DASH DIET MEAL PREP FOR BEGINNERS

Lower Your Blood Pressure and Improve Your Health with Simple and Tasty Recipes

NICOLE A. HARRIS

Table Of Contents

Whole Wheat Breakfast Burritos with Scrambled Eggs and Turkey Bacon

Veggie Breakfast Casserole with Hash Browns and Peppers

Oatmeal with Sliced Bananas and Honey

Breakfast Quesadillas with Scrambled Eggs, Cheese, and Salsa

Shakshuka with Poached Eggs in Tomato Sauce

Spinach and Cheese Breakfast Muffins

Peanut Butter and Banana Smoothie with Almond Milk

French Toast with Fresh Berries and Maple Syrup

Breakfast Hash with Sweet Potatoes, Turkey Sausage, and Eggs

Apple Cinnamon Baked Oatmeal

Breakfast Sandwiches with Turkey Sausage Patties and Avocado

Chapter 3: Lunchtime Delicacies

Chicken Caesar Wrap with Caesar Dressing and Romaine Lettuce

Falafel Salad with Hummus Dressing

Grilled Vegetable Panini with Pesto and Mozzarella

Lentil and Chickpea Salad with Lemon-Tahini Dressing

Turkey and Cranberry Sandwich with Spinach and Cream Cheese

Black Bean and Corn Quesadillas with Guacamole

Tabbouleh Salad with Quinoa and Fresh Herbs

Chicken Shawarma Bowl with Tzatziki Sauce and Pita Bread

Greek Orzo Salad with Cucumber, Tomato, and Feta

Vegetable and Tofu Stir-Fry with Teriyaki Sauce

Moroccan Chickpea Stew with Couscous

BBQ Chicken Salad with Avocado and Corn

Caprese Panzanella Salad with Crusty Bread and Balsamic Glaze

Thai Peanut Noodle Salad with Crunchy Vegetables

Chicken and Hummus Wrap with Lettuce and Tomato

Chapter 4: Dinner Delights

Lemon Garlic Herb Grilled Chicken with Roasted Potatoes

Spicy Beef and Vegetable Stir-Fry with Brown Rice

Herb-Crusted Baked Tilapia with Quinoa Pilaf

Mushroom and Spinach Stuffed Chicken Breast

Vegetable Curry with Basmati Rice

Baked Zucchini Boats with Marinara Sauce and Ground

Beef and Vegetable Kebabs with Tzatziki Sauce

Honey Mustard Glazed Salmon with Steamed Broccoli

Stuffed Bell Peppers with Ground Beef and Rice

Chicken and Vegetable Skewers with Garlic Yoghurt Sauce

Moroccan Spiced Lamb with Couscous

Spinach and Ricotta Stuffed Pasta Shells

Grilled Portobello Mushrooms with Balsamic Glaze
Quinoa and Black Bean Enchiladas with Red Sauce
Lemon Herb Grilled Shrimp with Quinoa Salad

Chapter 5: Soups Sensations

Minestrone Soup
Vegetable Lentil Soup
Chicken and Vegetable Soup
Tomato Basil Soup
Creamy Butternut Squash Soup
Black Bean Soup
Spinach and White Bean Soup
Broccoli Cheddar Soup
Turkey and Vegetable Chilli Soup
Mushroom Barley Soup

Chapter 6: Snack Attack

Fruit Salad with Mint and Lime
Hummus and Pita Bread
Greek Yoghurt with Honey and Almonds
Ants on a Log (Celery with Peanut Butter and Raisins)
Edamame with Sea Salt
Popcorn with Olive Oil and Parmesan Cheese
Cucumber Slices with Cream Cheese and Dill
Almond Butter and Banana Rice Cakes
Trail Mix with Dried Fruit and Nuts
Greek Yoghurt Dip with Sliced Vegetables
Baked Sweet Potato Fries with Spicy Ketchup
Cherry Tomatoes with Mozzarella Balls and Basil
Apple Slices with Cinnamon and Almond Butter

Cauliflower Crust Margherita Pizza with Fresh Basil

Chickpea and Spinach Curry with Basmati Rice

Baked Eggplant Parmesan Stacks with Tomato Sauce and Mozzarella

Lemon Garlic Shrimp Pasta with Whole Wheat Linguine

Turkey Meatball Subs with Whole Wheat Hoagie Rolls and Marinara Sauce

Moroccan Vegetable Tagine with Couscous

Conclusion

Introduction

In the kitchen, where stories of love, care, and healing often unfold, this cookbook finds its roots in a heartfelt journey of familial connection and well-being, all centred around the Dietary Approaches to Stop Hypertension (DASH diet).

I embarked on this culinary exploration with a profound purpose – a mission born from a poignant chapter in my own family's narrative.

When a beloved family member was diagnosed with high blood pressure, a wave of concern and determination swept through our household.

It wasn't just about adapting to a dietary change; it was about crafting meals that not only nurtured the body but also spoke to the soul, in alignment with the DASH diet's focus on reducing sodium intake and emphasizing whole foods rich in nutrients.

This family member, who had always revelled in the joy of savouring delicious and flavourful dishes, faced a new reality where taste and health seemed at odds.

In response to this challenge, I became a culinary ally, stepping into the kitchen with a fervent commitment to proving that health-conscious meals need not compromise on taste.

Each recipe in this book is a testament to the belief that food can be both a source of nourishment and a celebration of flavour, all while adhering to the principles of the DASH diet.

As we navigated this culinary journey together, experimenting with ingredients, flavours, and techniques, it became clear that a dash of flavour, a sprinkle of creativity, and a dash of love could transform our family meals into a vibrant palette of healthful delights, in line with the DASH diet's goal of promoting heart health and reducing hypertension.

It is with immense joy and a deep sense of purpose that I share these recipes with you, hoping that they bring not just nourishment to your table but also the unmistakable joy that comes from savouring meals made with love and care, all while staying true to the principles of the DASH diet.

In the pages of this cookbook, you'll discover a treasure trove of recipes meticulously crafted to embody the core principles of the DASH diet – an eating plan renowned for its ability to reduce blood pressure, promote heart health, and foster overall wellness.

Embracing a philosophy that champions whole foods, fruits, vegetables, lean proteins, and low-fat dairy products while minimizing sodium and unhealthy fats, each recipe serves as a testament to the transformative power of mindful eating.

Beyond the mere act of preparing meals, DASH diet meal prep represents a commitment – a pledge to prioritize self-care and nurture our bodies with intentionality and compassion. It's about harnessing the inherent goodness of fresh, wholesome ingredients and infusing each dish with vibrant flavours and comforting aromas that elevate the act of nourishment into an art form.

Whether you're embarking on this culinary journey to support your own health goals or seeking to cultivate a more wholesome lifestyle for yourself and your loved ones, you'll find an abundance of inspiration within these pages.

From hearty breakfasts to satisfying dinners and delectable desserts, each recipe is thoughtfully curated to offer a harmonious balance of nutritional excellence and culinary delight.

So, as you embark on this voyage of culinary exploration, may you find joy in the simple pleasures of preparing wholesome meals, savouring each bite mindfully, and embracing the transformative potential of the DASH diet.

Here's to a future filled with vitality, nourishment, and a deeper connection to the food we eat and the lives we lead.

Chapter 1: Getting Started With DASH Diet

Embarking on a journey to embrace the DASH diet through meal preparation marks a significant step towards prioritizing health and wellness.

The DASH (Dietary Approaches to Stop Hypertension) diet is renowned for its effectiveness in lowering blood pressure and reducing the risk of chronic diseases such as heart disease and stroke.

However, like any lifestyle change, transitioning to the DASH diet requires careful planning and preparation.

Getting started with DASH diet meal prep involves understanding the principles of the diet and learning how to incorporate them into daily meal planning. At its core, the DASH diet emphasizes consuming nutrient-rich foods such as fruits, vegetables, whole grains, lean proteins, and low-fat dairy while limiting sodium, saturated fats, and added sugars. By focusing on these wholesome and balanced food choices, individuals can not only manage their blood pressure but also improve overall health and well-being.

Meal preparation plays a crucial role in the success of the DASH diet journey by promoting consistency and convenience. By dedicating time to plan and prepare meals in advance, individuals can avoid the temptation of unhealthy options and ensure that nutritious choices are readily available. Additionally, meal prepping allows for better portion control, making it easier to adhere to recommended serving sizes and avoid overeating.

Moreover, by incorporating a variety of flavourful recipes and meal ideas into the DASH diet meal prep routine, individuals can enjoy a diverse and satisfying culinary experience while reaping the health benefits of the diet.

Whether it's hearty breakfasts, flavourful stir-fries, or nourishing soups, there are endless possibilities to explore within the realm of DASH diet meal prep.

In essence, getting started with DASH diet meal prep sets the foundation for long-term success in adopting a healthier lifestyle. By prioritizing nutritious food choices, practising portion control, and embracing the convenience of meal preparation, individuals can take proactive steps towards achieving their health and wellness goals while adhering to the principles of the DASH diet.

What is the DASH Diet?

In the quest for optimal health and vitality, the DASH (Dietary Approaches to Stop Hypertension) diet stands as a beacon of balanced nutrition and holistic well-being.

Rooted in scientific research and endorsed by health professionals worldwide, the DASH diet offers a comprehensive approach to managing blood pressure, improving cardiovascular health, and promoting overall wellness.

The DASH diet is an evidence-based eating plan designed to reduce high blood pressure. It emphasizes the consumption of nutrient-dense foods rich in essential vitamins, minerals, and antioxidants while limiting the intake of sodium, saturated fats, and refined sugars.

By prioritizing whole grains, lean proteins, fruits, and vegetables, the DASH diet provides a foundation for a nourished body and a fortified immune system.

The benefits of adopting the DASH diet are manifold, extending beyond blood pressure management to encompass various aspects of health and well-being. Numerous studies have demonstrated the effectiveness of the DASH diet in reducing hypertension and lowering the risk of cardiovascular diseases, including heart attacks and strokes.

Furthermore, the DASH diet has been associated with weight loss, improved insulin sensitivity, and a reduced risk of developing type 2 diabetes.

One of the most remarkable aspects of the DASH diet is its ability to deliver these health benefits without sacrificing flavour or satisfaction. Unlike restrictive fad diets that leave individuals feeling deprived and unsatisfied, the DASH diet embraces a diverse array of delicious and wholesome foods. From vibrant breakfast bursting with colour and flavour to hearty soups brimming with nourishing ingredients, the DASH diet offers a tantalizing culinary journey that delights the palate while nourishing the body.

The DASH diet represents a paradigm shift in our approach to nutrition and health, offering a sustainable and enjoyable path to optimal well-being. By prioritizing whole foods, minimizing processed ingredients, and savouring the rich tapestry of flavours that nature has to offer, individuals can reap the benefits of improved health and vitality.

How the DASH Diet Helps Lower Blood Pressure

The Dietary Approaches to Stop Hypertension (DASH) diet has garnered significant attention for its effectiveness in lowering blood pressure and promoting overall cardiovascular health. This dietary pattern emphasizes the consumption of nutrient-rich foods, particularly fruits, vegetables, whole grains, lean proteins, and low-fat dairy products, while limiting the intake of sodium, saturated fats, and added sugars.

One of the key mechanisms by which the DASH diet lowers blood pressure is its focus on reducing sodium intake. Excessive sodium consumption is known to contribute to high blood pressure by causing the body to retain water, thereby increasing blood volume and putting strain on the cardiovascular system. By emphasizing whole, minimally processed foods and limiting the consumption of high-sodium processed foods and condiments, the DASH diet helps to reduce overall sodium intake, thereby supporting healthy blood pressure levels.

Moreover, the DASH diet is rich in potassium, magnesium, and calcium, which are essential minerals known to play a role in blood pressure regulation. Potassium, in particular, helps to counteract the effects of sodium by promoting the excretion of excess sodium through the urine. Additionally, the high fibre content of the DASH diet may also contribute to its blood pressure-lowering effects by improving cholesterol levels and promoting heart health. Overall, the combination of nutrient-rich foods and reduced sodium intake in the DASH diet makes it a valuable tool for managing hypertension and reducing the risk of cardiovascular disease.

Key Benefits of the DASH Diet

The DASH diet offers a myriad of health benefits, particularly in promoting heart health and reducing the risk of hypertension. Emphasizing the consumption of nutrient-rich foods like fruits, vegetables, whole grains, lean proteins, and low-fat dairy products, while limiting sodium, saturated fats, and added sugars intake, the DASH diet stands as a powerful dietary approach.

Primarily, the DASH diet is renowned for its ability to lower blood pressure. Studies consistently show significant reductions in both systolic and diastolic blood pressure levels, even without medication. By prioritizing foods rich in potassium, magnesium, and calcium, while reducing sodium intake, this dietary pattern maintains healthy blood pressure levels, enhancing cardiovascular health.

In addition to blood pressure management, the DASH diet boasts numerous other health benefits. These include:

Improved Heart Health: By emphasizing nutrient-rich foods and limiting sodium and saturated fats, the DASH diet promotes heart health and reduces the risk of cardiovascular diseases such as heart attacks and strokes.

Better Cholesterol Levels: Following the DASH diet can lead to improvements in cholesterol levels, specifically by reducing LDL (bad) cholesterol and triglycerides while increasing HDL (good) cholesterol.

Weight Management: The DASH diet encourages the consumption of whole, unprocessed foods and emphasizes portion control, which can support weight loss and weight maintenance goals.

Enhanced Nutrient Intake: With its focus on fruits, vegetables, whole grains, lean proteins, and low-fat dairy products, the DASH diet provides a wide array of essential nutrients, vitamins, and minerals necessary for overall health and well-being.

Reduced Risk of Chronic Diseases: By promoting a balanced and nutritious eating pattern, the DASH diet may help reduce the risk of chronic diseases such as type 2 diabetes, certain cancers, and osteoporosis.

Flexibility and Adaptability: The DASH diet can be tailored to individual preferences and dietary needs, making it suitable for a wide range of individuals, including those with food allergies, intolerances, or specific cultural or lifestyle preferences.

Long-Term Sustainability: With its emphasis on whole, unprocessed foods and portion control, the DASH diet offers a sustainable approach to eating that can be maintained over the long term, promoting lifelong health and wellness.

Overall, the DASH diet provides a balanced and nutritious eating pattern that offers numerous health benefits, making it a popular choice for individuals looking to improve their overall health and well-being.

Setting Realistic Goals

Setting realistic goals is crucial for success in any endeavour. Start by outlining your goals in detail and making sure they are SMART (specific, measurable, achievable, relevant, and time-bound). Consider your capabilities, resources, and priorities when setting goals to ensure they are attainable within your constraints.

Break larger goals into smaller, manageable tasks to maintain motivation and track progress effectively. Flexibility is key; be prepared to adjust your goals as circumstances change or new information arises. Celebrate achievements along the way, no matter how small, and learn from setbacks to continuously refine your approach. By setting realistic goals, you set yourself up for sustainable progress and long-term success.

Basics of Meal Prepping

Meal prepping is a strategic approach to food preparation that involves planning, cooking, and portioning meals ahead of time to streamline the process of eating throughout the week.

At its core, meal prepping revolves around the principle of efficiency, enabling individuals to save time, money, and energy while maintaining a nutritious diet. By dedicating a few hours to meal prepping each week, individuals can alleviate the stress and uncertainty associated with mealtime decisions, ensuring that healthy options are readily available even during hectic schedules.

The basics of meal prepping begin with careful planning. This involves selecting recipes, creating a grocery list, and allocating time for cooking and assembly. Once the ingredients are gathered, the cooking process begins, with meals often prepared in large batches to yield multiple servings.

Portioning is a crucial step in meal prepping, as it allows for easy storage and portion control, promoting balanced eating habits. Meals can then be stored in airtight containers in the refrigerator or freezer until ready to eat.

For adherents of the DASH diet, meal prepping takes on added significance. The DASH (Dietary Approaches to Stop Hypertension) diet emphasizes the consumption of fruits, vegetables, whole grains, lean proteins, and low-fat dairy while limiting sodium, saturated fats, and added sugars. By meal prepping in accordance with DASH principles, individuals can ensure that their meals align with the recommended nutrient intake and contribute to better management of blood pressure and overall cardiovascular health.

This proactive approach to meal planning empowers individuals to make healthier choices consistently, ultimately supporting their long-term well-being.

Essential Tools and Ingredients

In embarking on the journey of DASH diet meal preparation, understanding the requisite tools and ingredients is paramount.

A well-equipped kitchen serves as the foundation for efficient and enjoyable meal prep. Key tools include a sharp chef's knife for precise chopping, cutting boards for safe food preparation, and measuring cups and spoons for accurate ingredient portions.

Additionally, having versatile cookware such as pots, pans, and baking sheets ensures versatility in cooking methods.

Equally crucial are the ingredients that form the basis of DASH diet meals. Whole grains like quinoa, brown rice, and whole wheat pasta provide fibre and essential nutrients. Lean proteins such as chicken breast, turkey, fish, and legumes contribute to satiety and muscle maintenance.

A rainbow of fresh fruits and vegetables offers a variety of vitamins, minerals, and antioxidants to support overall health. Healthy fats like olive oil, avocado, and nuts provide flavour and promote heart health.

Stocking a pantry with staple ingredients like herbs, spices, canned beans, and low-sodium broths allows for endless culinary creativity while adhering to DASH diet principles. By arming oneself with these essential tools and ingredients, embarking on the journey of DASH diet meal preparation becomes not only achievable but also enjoyable and rewarding.

Grocery Shopping Tips for DASH Diet Success

Effective grocery shopping is crucial for success on the DASH diet, ensuring you have the right ingredients on hand to create nutritious and balanced meals. Here are some professional and comprehensive tips to streamline your grocery shopping experience while adhering to the DASH diet principles:

1. Plan Ahead: Spend some time organizing your weekly meal plan before you go to the shopping store. Consider incorporating a variety of fruits, vegetables, whole grains, lean proteins, and low-fat dairy products into your meal plan.

2. Make a List: Compile a detailed shopping list based on your meal plan and any staple items you may need to restock. Organize your list by categories such as produce, dairy, protein, and pantry staples to ensure you don't overlook any items.

3. Read Labels: When selecting packaged foods, carefully read the nutrition labels to check for sodium content, added sugars, and saturated fats. Opt for products with lower sodium levels and minimal added sugars to align with DASH diet guidelines.

4. Shop the Perimeter: Focus on shopping the perimeter of the grocery store where fresh produce, lean proteins, and dairy products are typically located. This will help you prioritize whole, unprocessed foods and minimize exposure to unhealthy processed foods found in the inner aisles.

5. Buy in Bulk: Consider purchasing staple items such as whole grains, legumes, and frozen fruits and vegetables in bulk to save money and ensure you always have healthy options on hand.

6. Choose Seasonal Produce: Incorporate seasonal fruits and vegetables into your meal plan as they tend to be fresher, more flavourful, and often more affordable than out-of-season produce.

By following these tips, you can streamline your grocery shopping process and set yourself up for success on the DASH diet by consistently choosing nutritious, whole foods that support your health and well-being.

Portion Control and Serving Sizes

Portion control and serving sizes play a crucial role in maintaining a balanced and healthy diet. By managing the amount of food we consume at each meal, we can better control our calorie intake and ensure that we're meeting our nutritional needs without overindulging.

In the context of the DASH (Dietary Approaches to Stop Hypertension) diet, portion control is particularly important as it emphasizes the consumption of nutrient-rich foods while limiting the intake of sodium, saturated fats, and added sugars.

Adhering to appropriate portion sizes helps individuals following the DASH diet achieve and maintain a healthy weight, which is essential for managing blood pressure and reducing the risk of cardiovascular disease.

Understanding serving sizes is key to effective portion control. Many people underestimate the amount of food they eat, leading to unintentional overeating. By familiarizing ourselves with standard serving sizes and recommended portions for different food groups, we can make more informed choices about our meals and snacks.

Practising portion control doesn't mean depriving ourselves of our favourite foods. It's about moderation and balance. By enjoying smaller portions of higher-calorie foods while increasing our intake of fruits, vegetables, lean proteins, and whole grains, we can create a satisfying and nutritious eating plan that supports our overall health and well-being.

In summary, portion control and serving sizes are integral components of a healthy lifestyle, especially when following the DASH diet. By mastering portion control techniques and being mindful of serving sizes, individuals can better manage their weight, improve their dietary quality and reduce their risk of chronic diseases like hypertension and heart disease.

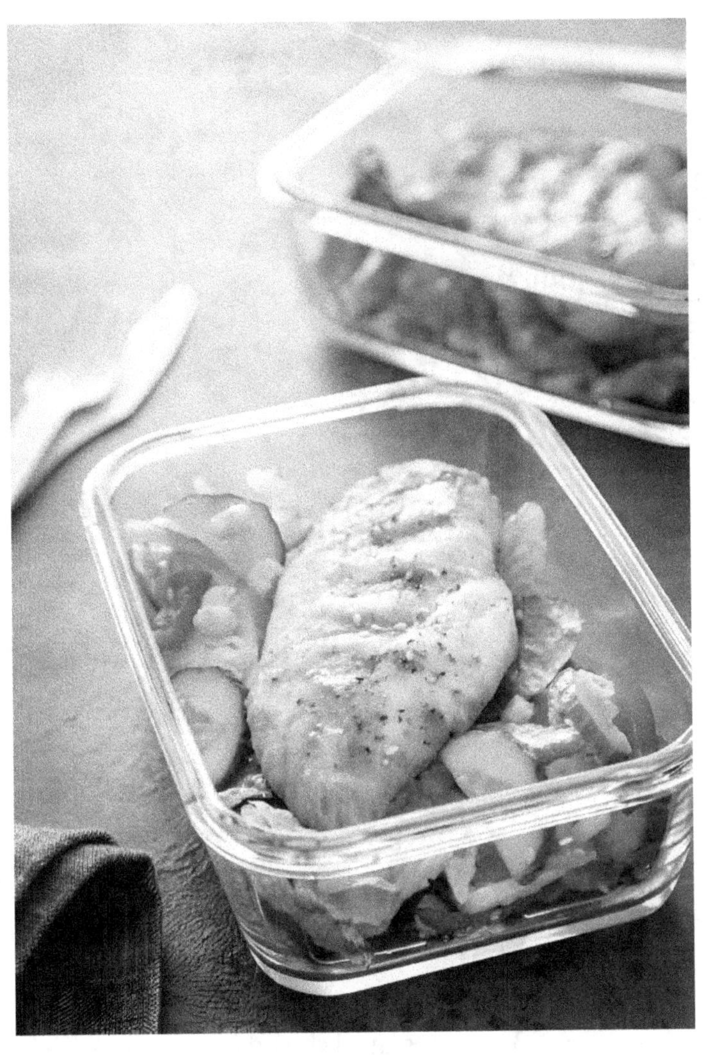

Chapter 2: Breakfast Boosters

Spinach and Feta Omelette

Preparation time: 5 minutes
Cooking time: 5 minutes
Servings: 1

Ingredients:
- 2 eggs
- 1/4 cup fresh spinach, chopped
- 2 tablespoons crumbled feta cheese
- Salt and pepper to taste
- 1 teaspoon olive oil

Directions:
1. In a bowl, whisk together the eggs, chopped spinach, crumbled feta cheese, salt, and pepper.
2. In a non-stick skillet, heat olive oil over medium heat.
3. Into the skillet, pour egg mixture and cook for 2-3 minutes until the edges start to set.
4. Gently lift the edges of the omelette with a spatula and tilt the skillet to allow any uncooked egg to flow underneath.

5. Once the omelette is mostly set but still slightly runny on top, fold it in half using the spatula.
6. Cook for another 1-2 minutes until the omelette is cooked through.
7. Allow the omelette to cool completely before storing it in an airtight container in the refrigerator.

Nutrition Value (per serving):
- Calories: 220 kcal
- Protein: 16g
- Carbohydrates: 2g
- Fat: 16g
- Fiber: 1g
- Sugar: 0g
- Sodium: 340mg

Mushroom and Swiss Cheese Omelette

Preparation time: 5 minutes
Cooking time: 10 minutes
Servings: 2

Ingredients:
- 4 large eggs
- 1 cup sliced mushrooms
- 1/2 cup shredded Swiss cheese
- Salt and pepper to taste

- 1 tablespoon olive oil or butter

Directions:

1. In a bowl, beat the eggs and season with salt and pepper.
2. Heat olive oil or butter in a non-stick skillet over medium heat.
3. Add sliced mushrooms to the skillet and sauté until tender.
4. Pour beaten eggs into the skillet, covering the mushrooms evenly.
5. Cook until edges are set, about 2-3 minutes.
6. Sprinkle shredded Swiss cheese over one-half of the omelette.
7. Fold the other half over the cheese.
8. Cook for another 2-3 minutes until cheese melts and eggs are cooked through.
9. Allow to cool before dividing into two portions and storing in meal prep containers.
10. Store in the refrigerator for up to 3-4 days.
11. To serve, reheat in the microwave until warmed through.

Nutrition Value (per serving):
- Calories: 250 kcal
- Protein: 18g
- Carbohydrates: 3g
- Fat: 18g
- Fiber: 1g

- Sugar: 1g
- Sodium: 300mg

Tomato and Basil Omelette

Preparation time: 5 minutes
Cooking time: 5 minutes
Servings: 1

Ingredients:
- 2 eggs
- 1 medium tomato, diced
- 2-3 fresh basil leaves, chopped
- Salt and pepper to taste
- 1 teaspoon olive oil

Directions:
1. In a bowl, whisk together the eggs, diced tomato, chopped basil, salt, and pepper.
2. In a non-stick skillet, heat olive oil over medium heat.
3. Into the skillet, pour the egg mixture and cook for 2-3 minutes until the edges start to set.
4. Gently lift the edges of the omelette with a spatula and tilt the skillet to allow any uncooked egg to flow underneath.

5. Once the omelette is mostly set but still slightly runny on top, fold it in half using the spatula.

6. Cook for another 1-2 minutes until the omelette is cooked through.

7. Allow the omelette to cool completely before storing it in an airtight container in the refrigerator.

Nutrition Value (per serving):
- Calories: 180 kcal
- Protein: 12g
- Carbohydrates: 4g
- Fat: 14g
- Fiber: 1g
- Sugar: 2g
- Sodium: 350mg

Blueberry and Almond Pancakes

Preparation time: 10 minutes
Cooking time: 10 minutes
Servings: 2

Ingredients:
- 1 cup all-purpose flour
- 1 tablespoon sugar
- 1 teaspoon baking powder
- 1/4 teaspoon salt

- 1/2 cup almond milk
- 1 egg
- 2 tablespoons melted butter
- 1/2 cup fresh blueberries
- 1/4 cup sliced almonds

Directions:

1. In a big mixing bowl, whisk together flour, baking powder, sugar, and salt.
2. In another bowl, beat the egg, then mix in almond milk and melted butter.
3. Pour wet ingredients into dry ingredients and stir until just combined (don't overmix).
4. Gently fold in blueberries and sliced almonds.
5. Heat a non-stick skillet or griddle over medium heat and lightly grease.
6. Pour 1/4 cup of batter onto the skillet for each pancake.
7. Cook for 2-3 minutes until bubbles form on the surface and the edges start to set.
8. Flip pancakes and cook for another 1-2 minutes until golden brown.
9. Repeat with remaining batter, greasing skillet as needed.
10. Allow pancakes to cool completely before storing them in an airtight container in the refrigerator.

Nutrition Value (per serving):
- Calories: 380 kcal
- Protein: 9g
- Carbohydrates: 42g
- Fat: 20g
- Fiber: 4g
- Sugar: 10g
- Sodium: 390mg

Veggie Scramble

Preparation time: 5 minutes
Cooking time: 10 minutes
Servings: 2

Ingredients:
- 4 eggs
- 1 cup mixed vegetables (such as bell peppers, onions, spinach)
- 1 tablespoon olive oil
- Salt and pepper to taste
- Optional toppings: grated cheese, chopped herbs

Directions:
1. In a non-stick skillet,heat olive oil over medium heat.

2. Add the mixed vegetables to the skillet and sauté for 3-4 minutes, or until they start to soften.
3. In a bowl, whisk the eggs together until well combined.
4. Over the sautéed vegetables in the skillet, pour the beaten eggs.
5. Cook, stirring occasionally, until the eggs are scrambled and cooked through, about 3-4 minutes.
6. Season with salt and pepper to taste.
7. Allow the veggie scramble to cool completely before dividing it into meal prep containers.
8. Optional: Sprinkle grated cheese or chopped herbs on top before storing.

Nutrition Value (per serving):
- Calories: 200 kcal
- Protein: 12g
- Carbohydrates: 5g
- Fat: 15g
- Fiber: 2g
- Sugar: 2g
- Sodium: 250mg

Banana Nut Muffins

Preparation time: 10 minutes

Cooking time: 20 minutes
Servings: 12 muffins

Ingredients:
- 2 cups whole wheat flour
- 1 teaspoon baking powder
- 1/2 teaspoon baking soda
- 1/4 teaspoon salt
- 3 ripe bananas, mashed
- 1/2 cup honey or maple syrup
- 1/4 cup unsweetened applesauce
- 2 eggs
- 1 teaspoon vanilla extract
- 1/2 cup chopped walnuts or pecans (optional)

Directions:
1. Preheat the oven to 350°F (175°C). Lightly grease a muffin tin with cooking spray or line with paper liners.
2. In a large mixing bowl, combine the whole wheat flour, baking powder, baking soda, and salt.
3. In another bowl, mash the ripe bananas until smooth. Add the honey or maple syrup, unsweetened applesauce, eggs, and vanilla extract. Stir until well combined.

4. Mix both the wet ingredients and the dry ingredients until thoroughly combined. Fold in the chopped nuts, if using.
5. Divide the batter evenly among the prepared muffin cups, filling each about 3/4 full.
6. Bake in the preheated oven until a toothpick inserted into the center of a muffin comes out clean or for 18 to 20 minutes.
7. Remove the muffins from the oven and allow them to cool completely in the tin before transferring them to an airtight container for storage.

Nutrition Value (per serving):
- Calories: 180 kcal
- Protein: 4g
- Carbohydrates: 30g
- Fat: 6g
- Fiber: 3g
- Sugar: 14g
- Sodium: 160mg

Greek Yogurt Smoothie Bowl

Preparation time: 5 minutes
Servings: 1

Ingredients:
- 1/2 cup plain Greek yogurt

- 1/2 cup frozen mixed berries
- 1 ripe banana, sliced
- 1 tablespoon honey
- 1/4 cup granola
- 1 tablespoon sliced almonds
- Optional toppings: additional fresh fruit, shredded coconut, chia seeds

Directions:

1. In a blender, combine the Greek yoghurt, frozen mixed berries, sliced banana, and honey.
2. Blend until smooth and creamy, adding a splash of water or almond milk if needed to reach your desired consistency.
3. Pour the smoothie into a bowl.
4. Top with granola and sliced almonds.
5. If desired, add additional toppings such as fresh fruit, shredded coconut, or chia seeds.
6. Cover the bowl with a lid or plastic wrap and store it in the refrigerator for up to 2 days.

Nutrition Value (per serving):

- Calories: 380 kcal
- Protein: 20g
- Carbohydrates: 55g
- Fat: 10g
- Fiber: 8g

- Sugar: 32g
- Sodium: 80mg

Greek Yogurt Parfait with Granola and Mixed Berries

Preparation time: 5 minutes
Servings: 2

Ingredients:
- 1 cup Greek yogurt
- 1/2 cup granola
- 1/2 cup mixed berries (such as strawberries, blueberries, and raspberries)
- Maple syrup or honey (optional, for drizzling)

Directions:
1. Divide the Greek yoghurt evenly between two meal prep containers.
2. Top each portion of yoghurt with 1/4 cup of granola.
3. Wash and dry the mixed berries, then divide them evenly between the containers.
4. Optionally, drizzle honey or maple syrup over the top for added sweetness.
5. Seal the containers and store them in the refrigerator for up to 3-4 days.

Nutrition Value (per serving):
- Calories: 200 kcal
- Protein: 12g
- Carbohydrates: 25g
- Fat: 6g
- Fiber: 4g
- Sugar: 10g
- Sodium: 60mg

Avocado and Egg Breakfast Bowl with Quinoa

Preparation time: 10 minutes
Cooking time: 15 minutes
Servings: 2

Ingredients:
- 1/2 cup quinoa
- 1 ripe avocado
- 2 eggs
- Salt and pepper to taste
- Optional toppings: diced tomatoes, sliced green onions, hot sauce

Directions:
1. Rinse the quinoa under cold water using a fine-mesh strainer. In a small saucepan, combine the quinoa with 1 cup of water. Bring to a boil, then reduce the heat to low,

cover, and simmer for 15 minutes, or until the quinoa is cooked and the water is absorbed. Take it off the heat and use fluff with a fork.

2. While the quinoa is cooking, prepare the avocado. Cut the avocado in half lengthwise then take out the pit. Scoop out the flesh and dice it into small pieces.

3. In a non-stick skillet, crack the eggs and cook them over medium heat to your desired doneness. Season with salt and pepper.

4. Divide the cooked quinoa between two meal prep containers. Top each container with half of the diced avocado and a cooked egg.

5. Let the meal prep containers cool for a few minutes before sealing them with lids and storing them in the refrigerator.

6. Optionally, store optional toppings like diced tomatoes, sliced green onions, or hot sauce separately in small containers to add before eating.

Nutrition Value (per serving):
- Calories: 330 kcal
- Protein: 13g
- Carbohydrates: 26g
- Fat: 20g
- Fiber: 7g
- Sugar: 1g

- Sodium: 80mg

Whole Wheat Breakfast Burritos with Scrambled Eggs and Turkey Bacon

Preparation time: 10 minutes
Cooking time: 15 minutes
Servings: 4

Ingredients:
- 4 whole wheat tortillas
- 6 eggs
- 4 slices turkey bacon, chopped
- 1/2 cup shredded cheddar cheese
- 1/4 cup diced tomatoes
- 1/4 cup diced bell peppers
- Salt and pepper to taste
- Optional toppings: salsa, avocado, Greek yoghurt

Directions:
1. In a non-stick skillet, cook the chopped turkey bacon over medium heat until crispy. Take them off the skillet and place aside.
2. In the same skillet, crack the eggs and scramble them over medium heat until cooked through. To taste, add salt and pepper for seasoning.

3. Warm the whole wheat tortillas in the microwave for 10-15 seconds to make them more pliable.
4. Divide the scrambled eggs, cooked turkey bacon, shredded cheddar cheese, diced tomatoes, and diced bell peppers evenly among the whole wheat tortillas.
5. Roll up each tortilla tightly, folding in the sides as you go to form a burrito shape.
6. Wrap each burrito individually in aluminium foil or parchment paper to keep them fresh.
7. Store the wrapped burritos in an airtight container in the refrigerator for up to 4 days.

Nutrition Value (per serving):
- Calories: 300 kcal
- Protein: 18g
- Carbohydrates: 22g
- Fat: 15g
- Fiber: 3g
- Sugar: 1g
- Sodium: 480mg

Veggie Breakfast Casserole with Hash Browns and Peppers

Preparation time: 15 minutes
Cooking time: 45 minutes
Servings: 6

Ingredients:

- 4 cups frozen hash browns, thawed
- 1 bell pepper, diced
- 1 onion, diced
- 1 cup diced tomatoes
- 1 cup chopped spinach
- 6 eggs
- 1/2 cup milk (or almond milk for a dairy-free option)
- 1 cup shredded cheddar cheese (or dairy-free cheese alternative)
- Salt and pepper to taste
- Optional: diced ham or cooked sausage for added protein

Directions:

1. Preheat your oven to 375°F (190°C). Lightly grease a 9x13-inch baking dish with cooking spray.
2. In a large mixing bowl, combine the thawed hash browns, diced bell pepper, diced onion, diced tomatoes, and chopped spinach. Mix well.
3. In a separate bowl, whisk together the eggs, milk, salt, and pepper.
4. Pour the egg mixture over the hash brown and vegetable mixture into the baking dish.

Gently stir to evenly distribute the ingredients.

5. Sprinkle the shredded cheese over the top of the casserole.
6. If desired, add diced ham or cooked sausage evenly over the top.
7. Cover the baking dish with aluminium foil and bake in the preheated oven for 30 minutes.
8. Remove the foil and bake for an additional 15 minutes, or until the eggs are set and the cheese is melted and bubbly.
9. Allow the casserole to cool completely before slicing it into individual portions.
10. Store the sliced portions in airtight containers in the refrigerator for up to 4 days.

Nutrition Value (per serving):
- Calories: 240 kcal
- Protein: 12g
- Carbohydrates: 18g
- Fat: 14g
- Fiber: 2g
- Sugar: 2g
- Sodium: 380mg

Oatmeal with Sliced Bananas and Honey

Preparation time: 5 minutes
Cooking time: 5 minutes
Servings: 1

Ingredients:
- 1/2 cup rolled oats
- 1 cup water
- 1 ripe banana, sliced
- 1 tablespoon honey

Directions:
1. In a small saucepan, bring water to a boil.
2. Stir in the rolled oats and reduce heat to low. Simmer for 3-5 minutes, stirring occasionally, until the oats are cooked to your desired consistency.
3. Remove the saucepan from the heat and allow the oatmeal to cool slightly.
4. Once cooled, divide the oatmeal into individual meal prep containers.
5. Top each portion with sliced bananas and drizzle with honey.
6. Seal the containers and store them in the refrigerator for up to 3-4 days.

Nutrition Value (per serving):

- Calories: 270 kcal
- Protein: 5g
- Carbohydrates: 57g
- Fat: 3g
- Fiber: 6g
- Sugar: 24g
- Sodium: 5mg

Breakfast Quesadillas with Scrambled Eggs, Cheese and Salsa

Preparation time: 10 minutes
Cooking time: 10 minutes
Servings: 2

Ingredients:
- 4 large eggs
- 1/2 cup shredded cheese (cheddar or Mexican blend)
- 4 small whole wheat tortillas
- 1/2 cup salsa
- Cooking spray or olive oil for greasing skillet

Directions:
1. In a bowl, beat the eggs until well scrambled.

2. Heat a non-stick skillet over medium heat and lightly grease with cooking spray or olive oil.

3. Pour the beaten eggs into the skillet and cook, stirring occasionally, until they are scrambled and cooked through. Remove from heat.

4. Place two tortillas on a clean surface. Divide the scrambled eggs evenly between the tortillas, spreading them out in an even layer.

5. Sprinkle shredded cheese over the scrambled eggs on each tortilla.

6. Top each tortilla with another tortilla to form a quesadilla.

7. Wipe the skillet clean and return it to medium heat. Lightly grease the skillet again.

8. Carefully transfer the quesadillas to the skillet and cook for 2-3 minutes on each side, or until golden brown and the cheese is melted.

9. Remove from heat and allow the quesadillas to cool completely before storing them in an airtight container in the refrigerator.

Nutrition Value (per serving):
- Calories: 390 kcal
- Protein: 22g

- Carbohydrates: 30g
- Fat: 20g
- Fiber: 5g
- Sugar: 3g
- Sodium: 780mg

Shakshuka with Poached Eggs in Tomato Sauce

Preparation time: 10 minutes
Cooking time: 20 minutes
Servings: 2

Ingredients:
- 1 tablespoon olive oil
- 1 small onion, diced
- 1 bell pepper, diced
- 2 cloves garlic, minced
- 1 can (14 oz) diced tomatoes
- 1 teaspoon ground cumin
- 1 teaspoon paprika
- Salt and pepper to taste
- 4 large eggs
- Fresh parsley, chopped (for garnish)

Directions:
1. In a skillet, heat olive oil over medium heat. Add diced onion and bell pepper, and cook until softened about 5 minutes.

2. Add in minced garlic and cook further for 1 minute.

3. Pour in the diced tomatoes (including juices) and stir in ground cumin, paprika, salt, and pepper. Simmer for 10 minutes, or until the sauce is somewhat thicker.

4. Using a spoon, make four wells in the tomato sauce. Crack an egg into each well.

5. Cover the skillet and let the eggs poach in the sauce for about 5-7 minutes, or until the egg whites are set but the yolks are still runny.

6. Remove from heat and garnish with chopped fresh parsley.

7. Allow the shakshuka to cool completely before dividing it into meal prep containers.

Nutrition Value (per serving):
- Calories: 210 kcal
- Protein: 12g
- Carbohydrates: 15g
- Fat: 13g
- Fiber: 4g
- Sugar: 8g
- Sodium: 470mg

Spinach and Cheese Breakfast Muffins

Preparation time: 10 minutes

Cooking time: 20 minutes
Servings: 6 muffins

Ingredients:
- 1 cup fresh spinach, chopped
- 1/2 cup shredded cheese (cheddar or mozzarella)
- 4 eggs
- 1/4 cup milk (any type)
- Salt and pepper to taste

Directions:
1. Preheat your oven to 350°F (175°C). Grease a muffin tin with cooking spray or line with paper liners.
2. Whisk the eggs and milk together thoroughly in a mixing bowl.
3. Stir in the chopped spinach and shredded cheese. To taste, season with salt and pepper.
4. Pour the mixture evenly into the prepared muffin tin, filling each cup about 3/4 full.
5. Bake in the preheated oven for 18-20 minutes, or until the muffins are set and lightly golden on top.
6. Allow the muffins to cool completely before storing them in an airtight container in the refrigerator.

Nutrition Value (per serving - 1 muffin):

- Calories: 100 kcal
- Protein: 8g
- Carbohydrates: 1g
- Fat: 7g
- Fiber: 0g
- Sugar: 0g
- Sodium: 150mg

Peanut Butter and Banana Smoothie with Almond Milk

Preparation time: 5 minutes
Servings: 2

Ingredients:

- 2 ripe bananas
- 2 tablespoons peanut butter
- 1 cup almond milk
- 1 tablespoon honey (optional)
- Ice cubes (optional)

Directions:

1. Peel the bananas and break them into chunks.
2. In a blender, combine the banana chunks, peanut butter, almond milk, and honey (if using).

3. Blend until smooth and creamy, adding ice cubes if desired for a colder smoothie.
4. Divide the smoothie between two airtight containers.
5. Seal the containers and store them in the refrigerator for up to 2 days.

Nutrition Value (per serving):
- Calories: 230 kcal
- Protein: 6g
- Carbohydrates: 25g
- Fat: 13g
- Fiber: 4g
- Sugar: 13g
- Sodium: 180mg

French Toast with Fresh Berries and Maple Syrup

Preparation time: 5 minutes
Cooking time: 10 minutes
Servings: 2

Ingredients:
- 4 slices whole wheat bread
- 2 eggs
- 1/4 cup almond milk
- 1 teaspoon vanilla extract

- 1/2 teaspoon cinnamon
- Cooking spray
- Fresh berries (such as strawberries, blueberries, or raspberries)
- Maple syrup

Directions:

1. In a shallow dish, whisk together the eggs, almond milk, vanilla extract, and cinnamon.
2. Dip each slice of bread into the egg mixture, coating both sides evenly.
3. Heat a non-stick skillet or griddle over medium heat and lightly grease with cooking spray.
4. Place the dipped bread slices onto the skillet and cook for 3-4 minutes on each side, or until golden brown and cooked through.
5. Remove the French toast from the skillet and allow it to cool completely before storing.
6. Once cooled, transfer the French toast to an airtight container, layering it with parchment paper if needed to prevent sticking.
7. Store the French toast in the refrigerator for up to 3-4 days.

Nutrition Value (per serving):
- Calories: 250 kcal
- Protein: 10g

- Carbohydrates: 40g
- Fat: 6g
- Fiber: 6g
- Sugar: 10g
- Sodium: 300mg

Breakfast Hash with Sweet Potatoes, Turkey Sausage, and Eggs

Preparation time: 10 minutes
Cooking time: 20 minutes
Servings: 4

Ingredients:
- 2 medium sweet potatoes, peeled and diced
- 8 ounces turkey sausage, sliced
- 1 bell pepper, diced
- 1 onion, diced
- 4 eggs
- Salt and pepper to taste
- 1 tablespoon olive oil

Directions:
1. Heat olive oil in a large skillet, over medium heat.
2. Add diced sweet potatoes to the skillet and cook until softened about 10 minutes.
3. Add turkey sausage, bell pepper, and onion to the skillet. Cook until sausage is browned

and vegetables are tender about 8-10 minutes.

4. In a separate skillet, fry or scramble eggs to your liking.
5. Divide the sweet potato and turkey sausage mixture into meal prep containers.
6. Top each container with a cooked egg.
7. Allow the containers to cool before sealing them and storing them in the refrigerator.

Nutrition Value (per serving):
- Calories: 320 kcal
- Protein: 20g
- Carbohydrates: 25g
- Fat: 15g
- Fiber: 4g
- Sugar: 6g
- Sodium: 480mg

Apple Cinnamon Baked Oatmeal

Preparation time: 10 minutes
Baking time: 30 minutes
Servings: 4

Ingredients:
- 2 cups old-fashioned oats
- 1 teaspoon baking powder
- 1 teaspoon ground cinnamon

- 1/4 teaspoon salt
- 2 cups almond milk
- 1/4 cup maple syrup
- 2 medium apples, diced
- 1/4 cup chopped nuts (optional)

Directions:
1. Preheat your oven to 375°F (190°C). Grease a baking dish with cooking spray or a little oil.
2. In a large mixing bowl, combine the oats, baking powder, cinnamon, and salt.
3. Add the almond milk and maple syrup to the bowl and mix well to combine.
4. Gently fold in the diced apples and chopped nuts (if using).
5. Pour the oatmeal mixture into the prepared baking dish, spreading it out evenly.
6. Bake in the preheated oven for 25-30 minutes, or until the oatmeal is set and the top is golden brown.
7. Remove from the oven and allow to cool completely before portioning into individual meal prep containers.
8. Store the baked oatmeal in the refrigerator for up to 4-5 days.

Nutrition Value (per serving):
- Calories: 250 kcal

- Protein: 6g
- Carbohydrates: 45g
- Fat: 6g
- Fiber: 6g
- Sugar: 18g
- Sodium: 200mg

Breakfast Sandwiches with Turkey Sausage Patties

Preparation time: 10 minutes
Cooking time: 15 minutes
Servings: 4

Ingredients:
- 4 whole wheat English muffins
- 4 turkey sausage patties
- 4 eggs
- 4 slices reduced-fat cheddar cheese
- Salt and pepper to taste

Directions:
1. Preheat your oven to 350°F (175°C).
2. Cook the turkey sausage patties according to package instructions. Set aside to cool.
3. In a non-stick skillet, fry the eggs over medium heat until cooked to your liking. Se
4. ason with salt and pepper.

5. While the eggs are cooking, split the English muffins and toast them in the oven for 5 minutes, or until lightly golden.

6. Once all components are cooked and cooled, assemble the sandwiches by placing one turkey sausage patty, one fried egg, and one slice of cheddar cheese on each English muffin.

7. Allow the sandwiches to cool completely before wrapping them individually in foil or plastic wrap.

8. Store the wrapped sandwiches in an airtight container in the refrigerator for up to 3-4 days.

Nutrition Value (per serving):
- Calories: 320 kcal
- Protein: 24g
- Carbohydrates: 26g
- Fat: 14g
- Fiber: 3g
- Sugar: 2g
- Sodium: 620mg

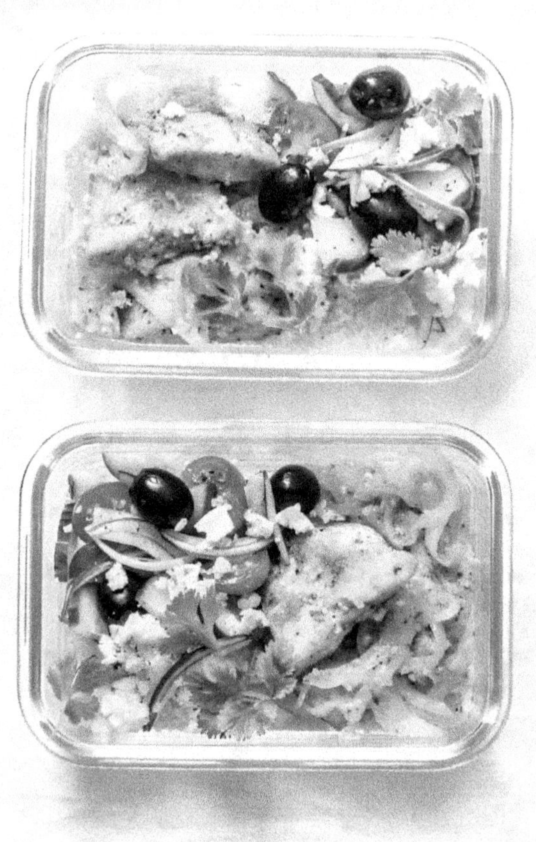

Chapter 3: Lunchtime Delicacies

Chicken Caesar Wrap with Caesar Dressing and Romaine Lettuce

Preparation time: 10 minutes
Cooking time: 10 minutes
Servings: 2

Ingredients:
- 2 large whole wheat tortillas
- 1 cup cooked sliced or shredded chicken breast
- 2 cups chopped romaine lettuce
- 4 tablespoons Caesar dressing
- 1/4 cup grated Parmesan cheese

Directions:
1. Lay out the tortillas on a clean surface.
2. Divide the cooked chicken evenly between the tortillas, placing it in the centre.
3. Top each tortilla with half of the chopped romaine lettuce.
4. Drizzle 2 tablespoons of Caesar dressing over each tortilla.
5. Sprinkle 2 tablespoons of grated Parmesan cheese over each tortilla.

6. Fold the sides of the tortillas towards the centre, then roll them up tightly into wraps.
7. Cut each wrap in half and place them in meal prep containers.
8. Seal the containers and store them in the refrigerator for up to 3-4 days.

Nutrition Value (per serving):
- Calories: 350 kcal
- Protein: 25g
- Carbohydrates: 25g
- Fat: 16g
- Fiber: 4g
- Sugar: 2g
- Sodium: 600mg

Falafel Salad with Hummus Dressing

Preparation time: 15 minutes
Cooking time: 20 minutes
Servings: 4

Ingredients:
- 1 can (15 oz) chickpeas, drained and rinsed
- 1/4 cup chopped fresh parsley
- 2 cloves garlic, minced
- 1 teaspoon ground cumin
- 1 teaspoon ground coriander
- 1/2 teaspoon salt

- 1/4 teaspoon black pepper
- 2 tablespoons olive oil
- 4 cups mixed salad greens
- 1 cucumber, diced
- 1 tomato, diced
- 1/4 cup diced red onion
- 1/4 cup hummus
- Juice of 1 lemon
- 2 tablespoons water

Directions:

1. Preheat your oven to 375°F (190°C).
2. In a food processor, combine the chickpeas, parsley, garlic, cumin, coriander, salt, and pepper. Pulse until the mixture is finely chopped and holds together when pressed.
3. Form the mixture into small patties or balls and place them on a baking sheet lined with parchment paper.
4. Drizzle the falafel patties with olive oil and bake for 20 minutes, flipping halfway through, until golden brown and crispy.
5. While the falafel is baking, prepare the salad ingredients. Divide the mixed salad greens, cucumber, tomato, and red onion among four meal prep containers.
6. In a small bowl, whisk together the hummus, lemon juice, and water to make the dressing.

7. Once the falafel is cooked, allow them to cool slightly before adding them to the meal prep containers.
8. Drizzle the hummus dressing over the salad and falafel.
9. Seal the meal prep containers and store them in the refrigerator for up to 4 days.

Nutrition Value (per serving):
- Calories: 290 kcal
- Protein: 10g
- Carbohydrates: 34g
- Fat: 14g
- Fiber: 9g
- Sugar: 5g
- Sodium: 470mg

Grilled Vegetable Panini with Pesto and Mozzarella

Preparation time: 10 minutes
Cooking time: 10 minutes
Servings: 2

Ingredients:
- 4 slices whole wheat bread
- 1/2 cup prepared pesto sauce
- 1 medium zucchini, sliced
- 1 red bell pepper, sliced

- 1/2 red onion, thinly sliced
- 4 slices mozzarella cheese
- Olive oil, for brushing

Directions:

1. Over medium heat, preheat a grill pan or panini press.
2. Brush the zucchini, bell pepper, and red onion slices with olive oil.
3. Grill the vegetables for 2-3 minutes on each side, or until tender and lightly charred.
4. Spread 2 tablespoons of pesto sauce onto each slice of bread.
5. Layer the grilled vegetables onto two slices of bread.
6. Top each sandwich with 2 slices of mozzarella cheese.
7. Place the remaining slices of bread on top to form sandwiches.
8. Place the sandwiches onto the grill pan or panini press.
9. Grill for 3-4 minutes on each side, or until the bread is toasted and the cheese is melted.
10. Remove from the grill and allow to cool completely before storing in an airtight container in the refrigerator.

Nutrition Value (per serving):

- Calories: 380 kcal

- Protein: 16g
- Carbohydrates: 35g
- Fat: 20g
- Fiber: 6g
- Sugar: 6g
- Sodium: 640mg

Lentil and Chickpea Salad with Lemon-Tahini Dressing

Preparation time: 10 minutes
Cooking time: 20 minutes
Servings: 4

Ingredients:
- 1 cup dried green lentils
- 1 can (15 ounces) chickpeas, drained and rinsed
- 1 red bell pepper, diced
- 1 cucumber, diced
- 1/4 cup chopped fresh parsley
- 1/4 cup chopped fresh mint
- Salt and pepper to taste

For the Lemon-Tahini Dressing:
- 1/4 cup tahini
- Juice of 1 lemon
- 2 tablespoons water
- 1 garlic clove, minced

- Salt and pepper to taste

Directions:
1. Rinse the lentils under cold water and place them in a saucepan. Cover with water and bring to a boil. Reduce heat to low, cover, and simmer for 15-20 minutes, or until the lentils are tender but still hold their shape. Drain any excess water and let the lentils cool.
2. In a large mixing bowl, combine the cooked lentils, chickpeas, diced bell pepper, diced cucumber, chopped parsley, and chopped mint.
3. In a small bowl, whisk together the tahini, lemon juice, water, minced garlic, salt, and pepper to make the dressing. If necessary, adjust the consistency by adding additional water.
4. Pour the lemon-tahini dressing over the lentil and chickpea mixture and toss until well coated.
5. Divide the salad into individual meal prep containers.
6. Seal the containers and store them in the refrigerator for up to 4 days.

Nutrition Value (per serving):
- Calories: 320 kcal

- Protein: 17g
- Carbohydrates: 40g
- Fat: 12g
- Fiber: 12g
- Sugar: 5g
- Sodium: 230mg

Turkey and Cranberry Sandwich with Spinach and Cream Cheese

Preparation time: 5 minutes
Cooking time: 0 minutes
Servings: 1

Ingredients:
- 2 slices whole wheat bread
- 2 ounces sliced turkey breast
- 1 tablespoon cream cheese
- 1 tablespoon cranberry sauce
- Handful of fresh spinach leaves

Directions:
1. Spread cream cheese on one slice of whole wheat bread.
2. Spread cranberry sauce on the other slice of bread.
3. Layer sliced turkey breast and fresh spinach leaves on top of the cream cheese.

4. Close the sandwich with the cranberry sauce side of the bread.
5. Cut the sandwich in half, if desired, and wrap it tightly in plastic wrap or place it in an airtight container.
6. Repeat for additional servings, if making more than one.
7. Store the sandwiches in the refrigerator until ready to eat.

Nutrition Value (per serving):
- Calories: 290 kcal
- Protein: 20g
- Carbohydrates: 35g
- Fat: 8g
- Fiber: 5g
- Sugar: 10g
- Sodium: 480mg

Black Bean and Corn Quesadillas with Guacamole

Preparation time: 10 minutes
Cooking time: 10 minutes
Servings: 2

Ingredients:
- 4 whole wheat tortillas
- 1 cup rinsed and drained canned black beans

- 1/2 cup frozen corn, thawed
- 1/2 cup shredded cheddar cheese
- 1 avocado, mashed
- 1 tablespoon lime juice
- Salt and pepper to taste
- Optional toppings: salsa, Greek yoghurt, cilantro

Directions:

1. In a bowl, mix together the black beans and corn. Set aside.
2. Spread mashed avocado evenly onto two of the tortillas.
3. Top the avocado-covered tortillas with the black bean and corn mixture, then sprinkle shredded cheese on top.
4. Place the remaining two tortillas on top to form quesadillas.
5. Heat a non-stick skillet over medium heat. Place one quesadilla in the skillet and cook for 3-4 minutes on each side, or until golden brown and the cheese is melted.
6. Repeat with the second quesadilla.
7. Allow the quesadillas to cool completely before slicing them into wedges.
8. Divide the quesadilla wedges into meal prep containers.
9. Store any optional toppings in separate containers to add before serving.

Nutrition Value (per serving):
- Calories: 450 kcal
- Protein: 18g
- Carbohydrates: 54g
- Fat: 20g
- Fiber: 12g
- Sugar: 3g
- Sodium: 610mg

Tabbouleh Salad with Quinoa and Fresh Herbs

Preparation time: 15 minutes
Cooking time: 15 minutes
Servings: 4

Ingredients:
- 1 cup quinoa
- 2 cups water
- 1 cup cherry tomatoes, halved
- 1 cucumber, diced
- 1/2 cup fresh parsley, chopped
- 1/4 cup fresh mint leaves, chopped
- 1/4 cup red onion, finely chopped
- 1/4 cup lemon juice
- 2 tablespoons olive oil
- Salt and pepper to taste

Directions:

1. Rinse the quinoa under cold water using a fine-mesh strainer. In a medium pot or saucepan, combine water and the quinoa. Bring to a boil, then reduce the heat to low, cover, and simmer for 15 minutes, or until the quinoa is cooked and the water is absorbed. Take it off from heat and let it cool.
2. In a large mixing bowl, combine the cooked quinoa, cherry tomatoes, cucumber, parsley, mint, and red onion.
3. Whisk the olive oil, lemon juice, salt, and pepper in a small bowl to create the dressing.
4. Pour the dressing over the salad and toss until well combined.
5. Divide the salad into individual meal prep containers and store them in the refrigerator for up to 4 days.

Nutrition Value (per serving):

- Calories: 250 kcal
- Protein: 6g
- Carbohydrates: 34g
- Fat: 10g
- Fiber: 5g
- Sugar: 3g
- Sodium: 120mg

Chicken Shawarma Bowl with Tzatziki Sauce and Pita Bread

Preparation time: 15 minutes
Cooking time: 20 minutes
Servings: 4

Ingredients:

- 1 lb boneless, skinless chicken breasts, sliced into strips
- 1 tablespoon olive oil
- 2 teaspoons ground cumin
- 2 teaspoons paprika
- 1 teaspoon garlic powder
- Salt and pepper to taste
- 4 pita bread rounds
- 1 cup Greek yogurt
- 1 cucumber, grated
- 1 clove garlic, minced
- 1 tablespoon lemon juice
- 2 tablespoons fresh dill, chopped
- 2 cups cooked brown rice
- 2 cups shredded lettuce
- 1 cup cherry tomatoes, halved
- 1/2 red onion, thinly sliced
- Optional toppings: sliced olives, chopped parsley, feta cheese

Directions:

1. In a bowl, toss the chicken strips with olive oil, ground cumin, paprika, garlic powder, salt, and pepper until evenly coated.
2. Heat a skillet over medium-high heat and cook the seasoned chicken strips for 6-8 minutes, or until cooked through and lightly browned. Remove from heat and set aside.
3. In another bowl, mix together the Greek yoghurt, grated cucumber, minced garlic, lemon juice, and chopped dill to make the tzatziki sauce.
4. Divide the cooked brown rice, shredded lettuce, cherry tomatoes, and sliced red onion evenly among four meal prep containers.
5. Top each container with the cooked chicken strips.
6. Divide the tzatziki sauce into small containers and add one container to each meal prep container.
7. Wrap the pita bread rounds in foil and store them separately.
8. Store the pita bread rounds separately, wrapped in foil, in the refrigerator until ready to eat.

Nutrition Value (per serving):
- Calories: 450 kcal
- Protein: 30g

- Carbohydrates: 40g
- Fat: 18g
- Fiber: 6g
- Sugar: 6g
- Sodium: 500mg

Greek Orzo Salad with Cucumber, Tomato, and Feta

Preparation time: 10 minutes
Cooking time: 10 minutes
Servings: 4

Ingredients:

- 1 cup orzo pasta
- 1 cucumber, diced
- 1 cup cherry tomatoes, halved
- 1/2 cup crumbled feta cheese
- 1/4 cup chopped fresh parsley
- 2 tablespoons extra virgin olive oil
- 2 tablespoons lemon juice
- Salt and pepper to taste

Directions:

1. As directed on the package, prepare the orzo pasta. To cool, empty and then rinse with cold water.
2. In a large mixing bowl, combine the cooked orzo pasta, diced cucumber, halved cherry tomatoes, crumbled feta cheese, and chopped fresh parsley.
3. Drizzle with extra virgin olive oil and lemon juice.
4. To taste, season with salt and pepper.
5. Toss everything together until well combined.
6. Divide the Greek Orzo Salad into meal prep containers.
7. Seal the containers and store them in the refrigerator for up to 3-4 days.

Nutrition Value (per serving):
- Calories: 250 kcal
- Protein: 8g
- Carbohydrates: 30g
- Fat: 10g
- Fiber: 3g
- Sugar: 3g
- Sodium: 200mg

Vegetable and Tofu Stir-Fry with Teriyaki Sauce

Preparation time: 10 minutes
Cooking time: 15 minutes
Servings: 2

Ingredients:
- 1 block of firm tofu, drained and cubed
- 2 cups mixed vegetables (such as bell peppers, broccoli, carrots, and snap peas), chopped
- 2 tablespoons teriyaki sauce
- 1 tablespoon olive oil
- Salt and pepper to taste
- Cooked brown rice or quinoa, for serving (optional)

Directions:

1. In a large skillet or wok, heat the olive oil over medium-high heat.
2. Add the cubed tofu to the skillet and cook for 5-6 minutes, or until lightly browned on all sides.
3. Add the mixed vegetables to the skillet and stir-fry for an additional 5-7 minutes, or until tender-crisp.
4. Pour the teriyaki sauce over the tofu and vegetables, and toss to coat evenly. Cook for another 1-2 minutes to heat through.
5. Remove the skillet from heat and let the stir-
6. fry cool completely.
7. Divide the stir-fry into meal prep containers, along with cooked brown rice or quinoa if desired.
8. Seal the containers and store them in the refrigerator for up to 3-4 days.

Nutrition Value (per serving without rice/quinoa):

- Calories: 220 kcal
- Protein: 16g
- Carbohydrates: 14g
- Fat: 10g
- Fiber: 5g
- Sugar: 7g
- Sodium: 450mg

Moroccan Chickpea Stew with Couscous

Preparation time: 10 minutes
Cooking time: 25 minutes
Servings: 4

Ingredients:
- 1 tablespoon olive oil
- 1 onion, diced
- 2 cloves garlic, minced
- 1 teaspoon ground cumin
- 1 teaspoon ground coriander
- 1/2 teaspoon ground cinnamon
- 1/4 teaspoon ground turmeric
- 1 can (15 ounces) chickpeas, drained and rinsed
- 1 can (14.5 ounces) diced tomatoes
- 2 cups vegetable broth
- 1 cup frozen peas
- Salt and pepper to taste
- 1 cup dry couscous
- Fresh cilantro, chopped, for garnish (optional)

Directions:

1. Heat olive oil in a big pot, over medium heat. Add diced onion and minced garlic. Cook until softened, about 5 minutes.
2. Add ground cumin, ground coriander, ground cinnamon, and ground turmeric to the pot. Stir well to evenly coat the onions and garlic with the spices.
3. Add chickpeas, diced tomatoes, and vegetable broth to the pot. Stir to combine.
4. Bring the mixture to a simmer and cook for 15 minutes, stirring occasionally.
5. Add frozen peas to the pot and cook for an additional 5 minutes, or until heated through.
6. While the stew is cooking, prepare the couscous according to package instructions.
7. Portion the Moroccan Chickpea Stew into meal prep containers over cooked couscous.
8. If desired, garnish each container with chopped fresh cilantro.
9. Seal the containers and refrigerate for up to 3-4 days.

Nutrition Value (per serving):
- Calories: 350 kcal
- Protein: 12g
- Carbohydrates: 60g
- Fat: 7g

- Fiber: 12g
- Sugar: 9g
- Sodium: 750mg

BBQ Chicken Salad with Avocado and Corn

Preparation time: 10 minutes
Cooking time: 15 minutes
Servings: 2

Ingredients:

- 2 boneless, skinless chicken breasts
- 1/2 cup fresh or frozen corn kernels
- 1 avocado, diced
- 4 cups mixed salad greens
- 1/4 cup BBQ sauce
- Salt and pepper to taste
- Optional toppings: sliced red onion, cherry tomatoes, shredded cheese

Directions:

1. Preheat the grill pan or grill over medium-high heat. Add salt and pepper to chicken breasts for seasoning.
2. Grill chicken for 6-7 minutes per side, or until cooked through and no longer pink in the center. Remove from heat and let cool.

3. While the chicken is cooking, heat a skillet over medium heat. Add corn kernels and cook for 3-4 minutes, or until lightly charred. Remove from heat and let cool.
4. Once cooled, slice the grilled chicken into bite-sized pieces.
5. In a large mixing bowl, combine the mixed salad greens, diced avocado, grilled chicken, and charred corn.
6. Drizzle BBQ sauce over the salad and toss gently to coat.
7. Divide the salad into two meal prep containers.
8. If desired, top each salad with optional toppings such as sliced red onion, cherry tomatoes, or shredded cheese.
9. Seal the containers and store them in the refrigerator for up to 3-4 days.

Nutrition Value (per serving):
- Calories: 350 kcal
- Protein: 30g
- Carbohydrates: 25g
- Fat: 15g
- Fiber: 8g
- Sugar: 7g
- Sodium: 420mg

Caprese Panzanella Salad with Crusty Bread and Balsamic Glaze

Preparation time: 10 minutes
Cooking time: 10 minutes
Servings: 4

Ingredients:
- 4 cups cubed crusty bread (such as ciabatta or sourdough)
- 2 cups cherry tomatoes, halved
- 1 cup fresh halved mozzarella balls (bocconcini)
- 1/4 cup fresh basil leaves, torn
- 2 tablespoons balsamic glaze
- Salt and pepper to taste
- Optional: extra virgin olive oil for drizzling

Directions:
1. Preheat the oven to 375°F (190°C).
2. Spread the cubed bread on a baking sheet and bake for 8-10 minutes, or until lightly toasted and crispy. Let it cool completely before storing.
3. In a large mixing bowl, combine the toasted bread cubes, cherry tomatoes, mozzarella balls, and torn basil leaves.
4. Drizzle the balsamic glaze over the salad and season with salt and pepper to taste. If

desired, drizzle with a little extra virgin olive oil.

5. Gently toss the salad until everything is well combined.
6. Divide the salad into individual meal prep containers.
7. Seal the containers and store them in the refrigerator for up to 2-3 days.

Nutrition Value (per serving):
- Calories: 250 kcal
- Protein: 10g
- Carbohydrates: 35g
- Fat: 8g
- Fiber: 3g
- Sugar: 5g
- Sodium: 450mg

Thai Peanut Noodle Salad with Crunchy Vegetables

Preparation time: 15 minutes
Cooking time: 10 minutes
Servings: 4

Ingredients:

- 8 oz rice noodles or whole wheat spaghetti
- 1 cup shredded cabbage
- 1 cup shredded carrots
- 1 red bell pepper, thinly sliced
- 1/2 cup chopped green onions
- 1/4 cup chopped cilantro
- 1/4 cup chopped peanuts (for garnish)

For the Peanut Dressing:

- 1/4 cup creamy peanut butter
- 2 tablespoons soy sauce
- 2 tablespoons rice vinegar
- 1 tablespoon honey or maple syrup
- 1 clove garlic, minced
- 1 teaspoon grated ginger
- 1 tablespoon lime juice
- 2-3 tablespoons water (to thin as needed)

Directions:

1. Cook the noodles according to package instructions. To halt the cooking process, drain and rinse well with cold water. Set aside.
2. In a large mixing bowl, combine the shredded cabbage, shredded carrots, sliced red bell pepper, chopped green onions, and chopped cilantro.

3. In a separate bowl, whisk together all the ingredients for the peanut dressing until smooth. If the dressing is too thick, add water, 1 tablespoon at a time, until the desired consistency is reached.
4. Pour the peanut dressing over the prepared vegetables and toss until evenly coated.
5. Divide the cooked noodles into meal prep containers. Top with the dressed vegetables.
6. Garnish each container with chopped peanuts.
7. Seal the containers and store them in the refrigerator for up to 4 days.

Nutrition Value (per serving):
- Calories: 380 kcal
- Protein: 12g
- Carbohydrates: 50g
- Fat: 16g
- Fiber: 8g
- Sugar: 8g
- Sodium: 450mg

Chicken and Hummus Wrap with Lettuce and Tomato

Preparation time: 10 minutes
Cooking time: 10 minutes
Servings: 2

Ingredients:

- 2 large whole wheat tortillas
- 1 cup shredded cooked chicken breast
- 1/2 cup hummus
- 1 cup shredded lettuce
- 1 tomato, thinly sliced

Directions:

1. Lay out the tortillas on a clean surface.
2. Spread a generous layer of hummus onto each tortilla, leaving about an inch border around the edges.
3. Divide the shredded chicken evenly between the two tortillas, spreading it out in a line down the centre of each.
4. Top the chicken with shredded lettuce and thinly sliced tomato.
5. Fold in the sides of each tortilla, then roll them up tightly from the bottom to create wraps.
6. Cut each wrap in half diagonally, if desired.
7. Store the wraps in an airtight container in the refrigerator until ready to eat.

Nutrition Value (per serving):

- Calories: 350 kcal
- Protein: 25g
- CarAbohydrates: 35g

- Fat: 12g
- Fiber: 8g
- Sugar: 3g
- Sodium: 550mg

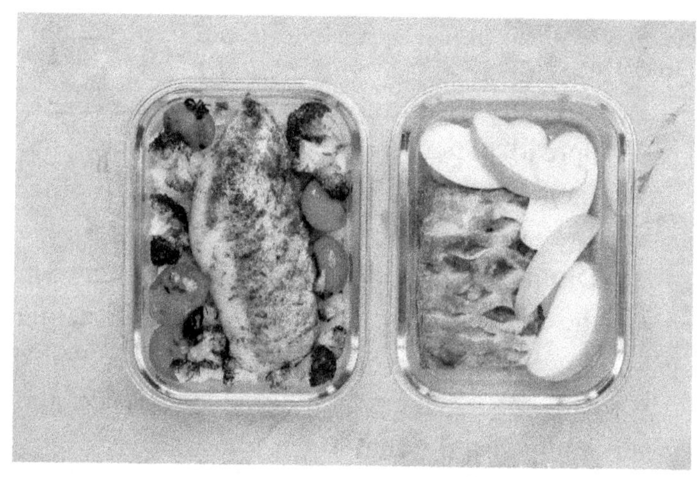

Chapter 4: Dinner Delights

Lemon Garlic Herb Grilled Chicken with Roasted Potatoes

Preparation time: 10 minutes
Cooking time: 30 minutes
Servings: 2

Ingredients:

- 2 boneless, skinless chicken breasts
- 2 tablespoons olive oil
- 2 cloves garlic, minced
- 1 tablespoon fresh lemon juice
- 1 teaspoon dried mixed herbs (such as thyme, rosemary, and oregano)
- Salt and pepper to taste
- 2 medium potatoes, cut into wedges

Directions:

- Preheat your grill pan or grill to medium-high heat.
- In a small bowl, mix together the olive oil, minced garlic, lemon juice, dried herbs, salt, and pepper.
- Place the chicken breasts in a shallow dish or resealable plastic bag and pour the marinade over them. Make sure the chicken is evenly coated. Allow to marinate for at

least 15 minutes, or overnight for the best flavor.

- While the chicken is marinating, preheat your oven to 425°F (220°C).
- Place the potato wedges on a baking sheet and drizzle with olive oil. Season with salt and pepper to taste. Toss to coat evenly.
- Roast the potatoes in the preheated oven for 25-30 minutes, or until golden brown and tender, flipping halfway through.
- While the potatoes are roasting, grill the chicken breasts for 6-8 minutes per side, or until cooked through and no longer pink in the center.
- Once cooked, remove the chicken from the grill and allow it to rest for a few minutes before slicing.
- Divide the grilled chicken and roasted potatoes into meal prep containers.
- Allow to cool completely before sealing the containers and storing them in the refrigerator.

Nutrition Value (per serving):
- Calories: 380 kcal
- Protein: 30g
- Carbohydrates: 25g
- Fat: 18g
- Fiber: 3g

- Sugar: 2g
- Sodium: 380mg

Spicy Beef and Vegetable Stir-Fry with Brown Rice

Preparation time: 15 minutes
Cooking time: 15 minutes
Servings: 4

Ingredients:
- 1 lb lean beef, thinly sliced
- 2 cups mixed vegetables (carrots, bell peppers, broccoli)
- 2 cloves garlic, minced
- 1 tablespoon ginger, minced
- 2 tablespoons low-sodium soy sauce
- 1 tablespoon sriracha sauce (adjust to taste)
- 1 tablespoon olive oil
- 2 cups cooked brown rice

Directions:
1. In a large skillet or wok, heat olive oil over medium-high heat.
2. Add minced garlic and ginger, and stir-fry for 30 seconds until fragrant.
3. Add thinly sliced beef to the skillet and cook until browned about 2-3 minutes.

4. Add mixed vegetables to the skillet and continue to stir-fry until they are tender-crisp about 3-4 minutes.

5. In a small bowl, mix together low-sodium soy sauce and sriracha sauce. Over the mixture of beef and vegetables in the skillet, pour the sauce.

6. Stir well to coat the beef and vegetables evenly with the sauce.

7. Serve the spicy beef and vegetable stir-fry over cooked brown rice.

8. Allow the stir-fry to cool completely before dividing it into meal prep containers.

9. Store in the refrigerator for up to 3-4 days.

Nutrition Value (per serving):
- Calories: 350 kcal
- Protein: 25g
- Carbohydrates: 30g
- Fat: 15g
- Fiber: 5g
- Sugar: 3g
- Sodium: 400mg

Herb-Crusted Baked Tilapia with Quinoa Pilaf

Preparation time: 10 minutes
Cooking time: 20 minutes

Servings: 2

Ingredients:
- 2 tilapia fillets
- 1/4 cup breadcrumbs
- 1 tablespoon chopped fresh herbs (thyme, parsley, or rosemary)
- 1 teaspoon olive oil
- Salt and pepper to taste
- 1 cup cooked quinoa
- 1/4 cup diced bell peppers
- 1/4 cup diced cucumber
- 2 tablespoons chopped fresh parsley
- 1 tablespoon lemon juice
- Lemon wedges for serving

Directions:
1. Preheat the oven to 400°F (200°C).
2. In a small bowl, mix together the breadcrumbs, chopped fresh herbs, olive oil, salt, and pepper.
3. Place the tilapia fillets on a baking sheet lined with parchment paper.
4. Spread the breadcrumb mixture evenly over the top of each tilapia fillet, pressing gently to adhere.
5. Bake the tilapia in the preheated oven for 15-20 minutes, or until the fish is cooked

through and the breadcrumb topping is golden brown and crispy.

6. In the meantime, prepare the quinoa pilaf. In a mixing bowl, combine the cooked quinoa, diced bell peppers, diced cucumber, chopped fresh parsley, and lemon juice. Toss to combine.

7. Divide the herb-crusted baked tilapia and quinoa pilaf evenly into meal prep containers. Allow to cool before sealing the containers. Place lemon wedges in separate compartments or small containers for squeezing over the fish before eating.

8. Once cooled, refrigerate the meal prep containers for up to 3-4 days.

Nutrition Value (per serving):
- Calories: 250 kcal
- Protein: 25g
- Carbohydrates: 20g
- Fat: 8g
- Fiber: 3g
- Sugar: 1g
- Sodium: 250mg

Mushroom and Spinach Stuffed Chicken Breast

Preparation time: 15 minutes

Cooking time: 25 minutes
Servings: 4

Ingredients:
- 4 boneless, skinless chicken breasts
- 1 cup sliced mushrooms
- 2 cups fresh spinach
- 1/2 cup shredded mozzarella cheese
- Salt and pepper to taste
- 1 tablespoon olive oil
- Optional: Italian seasoning or garlic powder for extra flavour

Directions:
1. Preheat the oven to 375°F (190°C).
2. Heat the olive oil in a pan over medium heat. Add the sliced mushrooms and cook until tender, for about 5 minutes.
3. Add fresh spinach to the skillet and cook until wilted, about 2 minutes. Season with salt and pepper to taste.
4. Make a horizontal slit in each chicken breast to create a pocket for the stuffing.
5. Stuff each chicken breast with the cooked mushrooms and spinach mixture. Sprinkle shredded mozzarella cheese on top.
6. Season the stuffed chicken breasts with salt, pepper, and optional Italian seasoning or garlic powder.

7. Place the stuffed chicken breasts in a baking dish and bake in the preheated oven for 20-25 minutes, or until the chicken is cooked through and no longer pink in the centre.
8. Allow the stuffed chicken breasts to cool slightly before storing them in an airtight container in the refrigerator.

Nutrition Value (per serving):
- Calories: 250 kcal
- Protein: 30g
- Carbohydrates: 3g
- Fat: 12g
- Fiber: 1g
- Sugar: 1g
- Sodium: 350mg

Vegetable Curry with Basmati Rice

Preparation time: 15 minutes
Cooking time: 25 minutes
Servings: 4

Ingredients:
- 1 cup basmati rice
- 2 cups water
- 1 tablespoon olive oil
- 1 onion, chopped
- 2 cloves garlic, minced

- 1 tablespoon curry powder
- 1 teaspoon ground cumin
- 1 teaspoon ground coriander
- 1/2 teaspoon turmeric
- 1 can (14 oz) diced tomatoes
- 1 can (14 oz) coconut milk
- 2 cups mixed vegetables (such as carrots, bell peppers, broccoli, and cauliflower), chopped
- Salt and pepper to taste
- Fresh cilantro, for garnish (optional)

Directions:

1. Rinse the basmati rice under cold water until the water runs clear. In a medium saucepan, combine the rice and water. Bring to a boil, then reduce the heat to low, cover, and simmer for 15 minutes, or until the rice is tender and the water is absorbed.
2. While the rice is cooking, heat olive oil in a large skillet over medium heat. Add chopped onion and minced garlic, and cook until tender, for approximately 5 minutes.
3. Stir in the curry powder, ground cumin, ground coriander, and turmeric, and cook for another minute until fragrant.
4. Add the diced tomatoes (with their juices), coconut milk, and mixed vegetables to the skillet. Stir to combine.

5. Bring the mixture to a simmer, then reduce the heat to low, cover, and cook for 10-15 minutes, or until the vegetables are tender.
6. Season the curry with salt and pepper to taste.
7. Divide the cooked basmati rice and vegetable curry into meal prep containers.
8. Allow the curry to cool completely before sealing the containers and storing them in the refrigerator.

Nutrition Value (per serving):
- Calories: 380 kcal
- Protein: 7g
- Carbohydrates: 40g
- Fat: 23g
- Fiber: 6g
- Sugar: 5g
- Sodium: 480mg

Baked Zucchini Boats with Marinara Sauce and Ground Turkey

Preparation time: 15 minutes
Cooking time: 25 minutes
Servings: 4

Ingredients:
- 4 medium zucchinis

- 1/2 pound lean ground turkey
- 1 cup marinara sauce
- 1/2 cup shredded mozzarella cheese
- Salt and pepper to taste
- Olive oil for drizzling

Directions:

1. Preheat your oven to 400°F (200°C).
2. Cut the zucchinis in half lengthwise and scoop out the seeds and flesh with a spoon, leaving about 1/4 inch shell.
3. In a skillet, cook the ground turkey over medium heat until browned and cooked through. Drain any excess fat.
4. Season the turkey with salt and pepper, then stir in the marinara sauce.
5. Place the zucchini halves in a baking dish, and cut side up.
6. Fill each zucchini half with the turkey mixture.
7. Sprinkle shredded mozzarella cheese on top of each zucchini boat.
8. Drizzle olive oil over the zucchini boats.
9. Bake in the preheated oven for 20-25 minutes, or until the zucchini is tender and the cheese is melted and bubbly.
10. Allow the zucchini boats to cool completely before storing them in an airtight container in the refrigerator.

Nutrition Value (per serving):
- Calories: 200 kcal
- Protein: 18g
- Carbohydrates: 10g
- Fat: 9g
- Fiber: 3g
- Sugar: 6g
- Sodium: 350mg

Beef and Vegetable Kebabs with Tzatziki Sauce

Preparation time: 15 minutes
Marinating time: 30 minutes
Cooking time: 10 minutes
Servings: 4

Ingredients:
- 1 pound lean beef, cut into cubes
- 1 bell pepper, cut into chunks
- 1 red onion, cut into chunks
- 1 zucchini, sliced
- 8 cherry tomatoes
- Salt and pepper to taste
- Wooden or metal skewers

For the Tzatziki Sauce:
- 1 cup Greek yogurt

- 1/2 cucumber, grated and squeezed to remove excess moisture
- 1 clove garlic, minced
- 1 tablespoon lemon juice
- 1 tablespoon chopped fresh dill or mint
- Salt and pepper to taste

Directions:
1. In a bowl, combine the beef cubes with salt, pepper, and any desired marinade. Let it marinate in the refrigerator for at least 30 minutes.
2. Meanwhile, prepare the tzatziki sauce by combining all ingredients in a bowl. Refrigerate until ready to use.
3. Preheat the grill or broiler to medium-high heat.
4. Thread the marinated beef cubes, bell pepper, red onion, zucchini, and cherry tomatoes onto skewers, alternating between ingredients.
5. Grill or broil the kebabs for 3-4 minutes on each side, or until the beef is cooked to your desired level of doneness and the vegetables are tender.
6. Remove the kebabs from the grill or broiler and let them cool completely.
7. Store the cooled kebabs in an airtight container in the refrigerator.

Nutrition Value (per serving):

- Calories: 250 kcal
- Protein: 25g
- Carbohydrates: 10g
- Fat: 12g
- Fiber: 2g
- Sugar: 5g
- Sodium: 200mg

Honey Mustard Glazed Salmon with Steamed Broccoli

Preparation time: 5 minutes
Cooking time: 15 minutes
Servings: 2

Ingredients:

- 2 salmon fillets
- 1/4 cup honey
- 2 tablespoons Dijon mustard
- 1 tablespoon olive oil
- Salt and pepper to taste
- 2 cups broccoli florets

Directions:

1. Preheat your oven to 400°F (200°C).

2. In a small bowl, mix together the honey and Dijon mustard to make the glaze.

3. Arrange the salmon fillets on a baking pan lined with parchment paper.

4. Brush the honey mustard glaze over the salmon fillets, coating them evenly.

5. Drizzle the olive oil over the salmon and season with salt and pepper.

6. Bake the salmon in the preheated oven for 12-15 minutes, or until cooked through and flaky.

7. While the salmon is baking, steam the broccoli florets until tender, about 5-7 minutes.

8. Once cooked, allow the salmon and broccoli to cool completely before dividing them into meal prep containers.

9. Store the meal prep containers in the refrigerator for up to 3-4 days.

Nutrition Value (per serving):
- Calories: 350 kcal
- Protein: 25g
- Carbohydrates: 25g
- Fat: 18g
- Fiber: 4g
- Sugar: 20g
- Sodium: 300mg

Stuffed Bell Peppers with Ground Beef and Rice

Preparation time: 15 minutes
Cooking time: 45 minutes
Servings: 4

Ingredients:

- 4 large bell peppers, any colour
- 1 pound lean ground beef
- 1 cup cooked brown rice
- 1 cup tomato sauce
- 1 teaspoon garlic powder
- 1 teaspoon onion powder
- Salt and pepper to taste
- Optional toppings: shredded cheese, chopped parsley

Directions:

1. Preheat the oven to 375°F (190°C).
2. Cut off the tops of the bell peppers and remove the seeds and membranes. Place the bell peppers upright in a baking dish.
3. Cook the ground beef until browned in a skillet over medium heat. Drain any extra fat.
4. In a large mixing bowl, combine the cooked ground beef, cooked brown rice, tomato

sauce, garlic powder, onion powder, salt, and pepper. Mix well.

5. Stuff each bell pepper with the ground beef and rice mixture, pressing down gently to pack it in.
6. Cover the baking dish with aluminum foil and bake for 30-35 minutes, or until the bell peppers are tender.
7. Remove the foil and sprinkle optional shredded cheese on top of each stuffed bell pepper. Return to the oven and bake for an additional 5-10 minutes, or until the cheese is melted and bubbly.
8. Allow the stuffed bell peppers to cool slightly before transferring them to meal prep containers.
9. Store the stuffed bell peppers in the refrigerator for up to 4 days.

Nutrition Value (per serving):
- Calories: 320 kcal
- Protein: 25g
- Carbohydrates: 25g
- Fat: 12g
- Fiber: 5g
- Sugar: 7g
- Sodium: 480mg

Chicken and Vegetable Skewers with Garlic Yogurt Sauce

Preparation time: 15 minutes
Marinating time: 30 minutes
Cooking time: 10 minutes
Servings: 4

Ingredients:

- 1 lb boneless, skinless chicken breasts, cut into bite-sized pieces
- 1 zucchini, sliced into rounds
- 1 red bell pepper, chopped into chunks
- 1 red onion, cut into chunks
- 8 cherry tomatoes
- Salt and pepper to taste
- Wooden or metal skewers

For the Garlic Yogurt Sauce:

- 1 cup Greek yogurt
- 2 cloves garlic, minced
- 1 tablespoon lemon juice
- Salt and pepper to taste

Directions:

1. If using wooden skewers, soak them in water for at least 30 minutes to prevent burning.

2. In a bowl, combine the chicken pieces with salt, pepper, and any desired herbs or spices for seasoning.
3. Thread the marinated chicken, zucchini slices, bell pepper chunks, onion chunks, and cherry tomatoes onto the skewers, alternating between ingredients.
4. In a separate bowl, mix together the Greek yoghurt, minced garlic, lemon juice, salt, and pepper to make the garlic yoghurt sauce. Adjust seasoning to taste.
5. Divide the skewers and garlic yoghurt sauce into meal prep containers.
6. Seal the containers and store them in the refrigerator for up to 3-4 days.

To Serve:
1. When ready to eat, preheat the grill or grill pan to medium-high heat.
2. Cook the skewers for 3-4 minutes on each side, or until the chicken is cooked through and the vegetables are tender and slightly charred.
3. Serve the chicken and vegetable skewers hot with a side of garlic yoghurt sauce for dipping.

Nutrition Value (per serving, including sauce):
- Calories: 240 kcal

- Protein: 30g
- Carbohydrates: 10g
- Fat: 8g
- Fiber: 2g
- Sugar: 5g
- Sodium: 180mg

Moroccan Spiced Lamb with Couscous

Preparation time: 10 minutes
Cooking time: 25 minutes
Servings: 4

Ingredients:
- 1 lb lamb, cubed
- 1 tablespoon olive oil
- 1 onion, diced
- 2 cloves garlic, minced
- 1 teaspoon ground cumin
- 1 teaspoon ground coriander
- 1/2 teaspoon ground cinnamon
- 1/4 teaspoon ground ginger
- 1/4 teaspoon ground paprika
- 1/4 teaspoon ground turmeric
- Salt and pepper to taste
- 1 cup couscous
- 1 1/4 cups chicken broth

- Chopped fresh cilantro for garnish (optional)

Directions:
1. Heat olive oil in a large skillet over medium heat. Add diced onion and minced garlic, and cook until softened.
2. Add cubed lamb to the skillet and cook until browned on all sides.
3. Stir in ground cumin, ground coriander, ground cinnamon, ground ginger, ground paprika, ground turmeric, salt, and pepper. Cook for another minute until fragrant.
4. Fill the skillet with chicken broth and bring to a boil.
5. Stir in couscous, cover, and remove from heat. Let it sit for 5 minutes until couscous is tender and liquid is absorbed.
6. Fluff the couscous with a fork and divide it evenly into meal prep containers. Add the Moroccan spiced lamb on top of the couscous.
7. If preferred, garnish each container with freshly chopped cilantro before sealing for refrigeration.

Nutrition Value (per serving):
- Calories: 380 kcal
- Protein: 25g
- Carbohydrates: 35g

- Fat: 15g
- Fiber: 3g
- Sugar: 2g
- Sodium: 430mg

Spinach and Ricotta Stuffed Pasta Shells

Preparation time: 15 minutes
Cooking time: 25 minutes
Servings: 4

Ingredients:
- 20 jumbo pasta shells
- 2 cups ricotta cheese
- 1 cup chopped spinach, fresh or frozen (thawed and drained)
- 1/2 cup grated Parmesan cheese
- 1 egg
- 1 teaspoon dried oregano
- 1 teaspoon garlic powder
- Salt and pepper to taste
- 2 cups marinara sauce

Directions:
- Preheat the oven to 350°F (175°C).
- Cook the jumbo pasta shells according to package instructions until al dente. Drain and set aside to cool.

- In a mixing bowl, combine the ricotta cheese, chopped spinach, Parmesan cheese, egg, dried oregano, garlic powder, salt, and pepper. Mix well until fully combined.
- Stuff each cooked pasta shell with the spinach and ricotta mixture.
- Spread a thin layer of marinara sauce on the bottom of a baking dish.
- Arrange the stuffed pasta shells in the baking dish.
- Pour the remaining marinara sauce over the top of the stuffed shells.
- Place foil over the baking dish and bake it for 20 minutes in the preheated oven.
- Remove the foil and bake for an additional 5 minutes, or until the sauce is bubbly and the pasta is heated through.
- Allow the stuffed pasta shells to cool completely before portioning into meal prep containers.

Nutrition Value (per serving):
- Calories: 450 kcal
- Protein: 25g
- Carbohydrates: 45g
- Fat: 18g
- Fiber: 5g
- Sugar: 7g
- Sodium: 800mg

Grilled Portobello Mushrooms with Balsamic Glaze

Preparation time: 10 minutes
Cooking time: 10 minutes
Servings: 2

Ingredients:
- 2 large Portobello mushrooms
- 2 tablespoons balsamic vinegar
- 1 tablespoon olive oil
- 2 cloves garlic, minced
- Salt and pepper to taste
- Fresh parsley for garnish (optional)

Directions:
1. Preheat the grill pan or grill to medium-high heat.
2. Clean the Portobello mushrooms by gently wiping them with a damp paper towel to remove any dirt.
3. In a small bowl, whisk together the balsamic vinegar, olive oil, minced garlic, salt, and pepper.
4. Brush the mushroom caps with the balsamic mixture, coating them evenly.

5. Place the mushrooms on the preheated grill, gill-side down, and cook for 4-5 minutes.
6. Flip the mushrooms and continue to cook for another 4-5 minutes, or until they are tender and grill marks appear.
7. Remove the mushrooms from the grill and let them cool completely.
8. Once cooled, store the mushrooms in an airtight container in the refrigerator.

Nutrition Value (per serving):
- Calories: 80 kcal
- Protein: 3g
- Carbohydrates: 7g
- Fat: 5g
- Fiber: 2g
- Sugar: 4g
- Sodium: 10mg

Quinoa and Black Bean Enchiladas with Red Sauce

Preparation time: 15 minutes
Cooking time: 25 minutes
Servings: 4

Ingredients:
- 1 cup quinoa, cooked
- 1 can (15 oz) drained and rinsed black beans

- 1 cup corn kernels fresh, frozen, or canned
- 1 cup shredded cheese (cheddar or Mexican blend)
- 8 small whole wheat tortillas
- 1 can (10 oz) of red enchilada sauce

Directions:
1. Preheat the oven to 375°F (190°C).
2. In a large mixing bowl, combine the cooked quinoa, black beans, corn kernels, and half of the shredded cheese. Mix well.
3. Pour a small amount of enchilada sauce into the bottom of a baking dish.
4. Place about 1/3 cup of the quinoa and black bean mixture onto each tortilla, roll it up and place it seam-side down in the baking dish.
5. Pour the remaining enchilada sauce over the top of the enchiladas, spreading it evenly.
6. Sprinkle the remaining shredded cheese over the top.
7. Cover the baking dish with foil and bake in the preheated oven for 20 minutes.
8. Remove the foil and bake for an additional 5 minutes, or until the cheese is melted and bubbly.
9. Allow the enchiladas to cool slightly before storing them in an airtight container in the refrigerator.

Nutrition Value (per serving):

- Calories: 450 kcal
- Protein: 18g
- Carbohydrates: 62g
- Fat: 15g
- Fiber: 10g
- Sugar: 4g
- Sodium: 840mg

Lemon Herb Grilled Shrimp with Quinoa Salad

Preparation time: 15 minutes
Cooking time: 10 minutes
Servings: 2

Ingredients:

- 1/2 lb shrimp, peeled and deveined
- 1 tablespoon olive oil
- 1 lemon, juiced and zested
- 1 teaspoon dried herbs (such as oregano, thyme, or rosemary)
- Salt and pepper to taste
- 1 cup cooked quinoa
- 1 cup cherry tomatoes, halved
- 1/2 cucumber, diced
- 2 tablespoons chopped fresh parsley
- Optional: crumbled feta cheese for serving

Directions:

1. In a bowl, toss the shrimp with olive oil, lemon juice, lemon zest, dried herbs, salt, and pepper until evenly coated.
2. Preheat the grill or grill pan to medium-high heat. If using skewers, thread the shrimp onto them.
3. Grill the shrimp for 2-3 minutes on each side, or until they are pink and opaque.
4. In a large mixing bowl, combine the cooked quinoa, cherry tomatoes, diced cucumber, and chopped parsley. Toss with a drizzle of olive oil and lemon juice, and season with salt and pepper to taste.
5. Divide the quinoa salad between two meal prep containers.
6. Once the grilled shrimp have cooled, remove them from the skewers and add them to the meal prep containers.
7. Optional: Top with crumbled feta cheese before serving.

Nutrition Value (per serving):
- Calories: 280 kcal
- Protein: 25g
- Carbohydrates: 23g
- Fat: 10g
- Fiber: 4g
- Sugar: 3g

- Sodium: 280mg

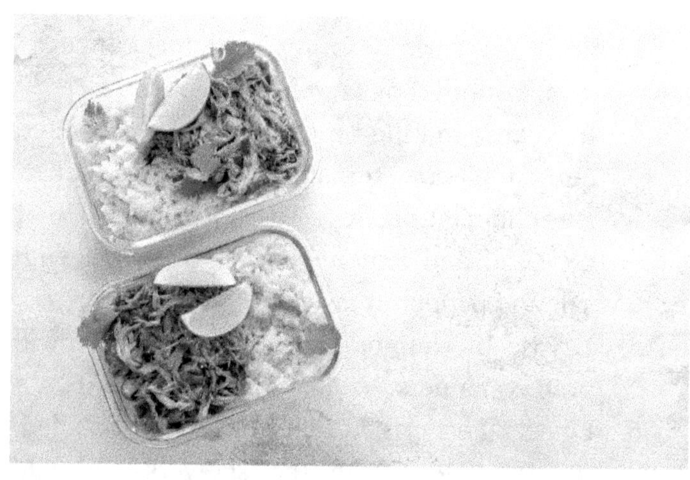

Chapter 5: Soups Sensations

Minestrone Soup

Preparation Time: 10 minutes
Cooking Time: 25 minutes
Servings: 6

Ingredients:

- 1 tablespoon olive oil
- 1 onion, diced
- 2 carrots, diced
- 2 celery stalks, diced
- 2 cloves garlic, minced
- 1 can (14 oz) diced tomatoes
- 4 cups vegetable broth
- 1 can (15 oz) kidney beans, rinsed and drained
- 1 can (15 oz) cannellini beans, drained and rinsed
- 1 cup chopped green beans
- 1 cup small pasta (e.g., macaroni or ditalini)
- 2 teaspoons dried oregano
- 1 teaspoon dried basil
- Salt and pepper, to taste
- Grated Parmesan cheese, for serving (optional)

Directions:

1. Heat olive oil in a large pot over medium heat.
2. Add diced onion, carrots, and celery to the pot. Cook until softened, about 5 minutes.
3. Stir in minced garlic and cook for another minute.
4. Add diced tomatoes, vegetable broth, kidney beans, cannellini beans, chopped green beans, pasta, oregano, and basil to the pot. Season with salt and pepper.
5. Bring the soup to a boil, then reduce the heat to low. Simmer for 15-20 minutes, or until the pasta and vegetables are tender.
6. Taste and adjust seasoning if needed.
7. Serve the minestrone soup in meal prep containers. Optionally, sprinkle with grated Parmesan cheese before sealing the containers.
8. Allow the soup to cool before storing it in the refrigerator or freezer.

Nutrition Value (per serving):
- Calories: 230 kcal
- Fat: 4g
- Carbohydrates: 39g
- Fiber: 9g
- Protein: 10g
- Sodium: 650mg

Vegetable Lentil Soup

Preparation Time: 10 minutes
Cooking Time: 25 minutes
Servings: 4

Ingredients:
- 1 cup green lentils, rinsed and drained
- 2 cups vegetable broth
- 1 tablespoon olive oil
- 1 onion, diced
- 2 carrots, diced
- 2 celery stalks, diced
- 2 cloves garlic, minced
- 1 teaspoon ground cumin
- 1 teaspoon ground coriander
- 1 teaspoon paprika
- Salt and pepper to taste
- Fresh parsley for garnish (optional)

Directions:
1. In a medium saucepan, combine the green lentils and vegetable broth. Bring to a boil, then reduce the heat and simmer for 20-25 minutes, or until the lentils are tender.
2. While the lentils are cooking, heat the olive oil in a large skillet over medium heat. Add the diced onion, carrots, and celery. Cook for about 5-7 minutes, or until the vegetables are tender.

3. Add the minced garlic, ground cumin, ground coriander, and paprika to the skillet. Cook for an additional 1-2 minutes, or until fragrant.

4. Once the lentils are cooked, add them to the skillet with the cooked vegetables. Stir well to combine. To taste, season with salt and pepper.

5. Divide the Vegetable Lentil Delight into meal prep containers. Garnish with fresh parsley if desired.

Nutrition Value (per serving):
- Calories: 250
- Protein: 12g
- Fat: 5g
- Carbohydrates: 40g
- Fiber: 10g
- Sugar: 6g
- Sodium: 500mg

Chicken and Vegetable Soup

Preparation Time: 15 minutes
Cooking Time: 30 minutes
Servings: 4

Ingredients:
- 1 tablespoon olive oil

- 1 pound diced, skinless, boneless, chicken breast
- 1 onion, diced
- 2 carrots, peeled and diced
- 2 celery stalks, diced
- 2 garlic cloves, minced
- 6 cups low-sodium chicken broth
- 1 bay leaf
- 1 teaspoon dried thyme
- Salt and pepper to taste
- 2 cups chopped spinach or kale
- Fresh parsley, for garnish (optional)

Directions:

1. Heat olive oil in a large pot over medium heat. Add diced chicken and cook until browned about 5 minutes.
2. Add diced onion, carrots, celery, and minced garlic to the pot. Cook, stirring occasionally, until vegetables are softened, about 5 minutes.
3. Pour in chicken broth and add bay leaf and dried thyme. Season with salt and pepper to taste.
4. Bring the soup to a boil, then reduce heat to low and let it simmer for 15-20 minutes until chicken is cooked through and vegetables are tender.

5. Stir in chopped spinach or kale and cook for an additional 5 minutes until wilted.
6. Remove the bay leaf from the soup and discard.
7. Allow the soup to cool completely before transferring it into meal prep containers.
8. Divide the soup evenly among the containers, leaving some space at the top for expansion during freezing or refrigeration.
9. Seal the containers tightly and store them in the refrigerator for up to 4 days or in the freezer for up to 3 months.
10. When ready to eat, reheat the soup in the microwave or on the stovetop until heated through.

Nutrition Value (per serving):
- Calories: 240
- Protein: 25g
- Fat: 8g
- Carbohydrates: 15g
- Fiber: 3g
- Sodium: 300mg

Tomato Basil Soup

Preparation Time: 10 minutes
Cooking Time: 25 minutes
Servings: 4

Ingredients:

- 6 ripe tomatoes, diced
- 2 cloves garlic, minced
- 1 small onion, finely chopped
- 2 cups low-sodium vegetable broth
- 1/4 cup fresh basil leaves, chopped
- 1 tablespoon olive oil
- Salt and pepper to taste

Directions:

1. Heat olive oil in a large pot over medium heat. Add minced garlic and chopped onion. Sauté until onions are translucent, about 3-4 minutes.
2. Add diced tomatoes to the pot and cook for another 5 minutes, allowing them to soften.
3. Pour in vegetable broth and bring the mixture to a simmer. Let it cook for 15 minutes, allowing the flavours to meld together.
4. Using an immersion blender or regular blender, blend the soup until smooth.
5. Stir in chopped basil leaves and season with salt and pepper to taste.
6. Divide the soup into four individual meal prep containers.

7. Allow the soup to cool completely before covering and refrigerating for up to 3-4 days.

Nutrition Value (per serving):
- Calories: 90 kcal
- Fat: 3g
- Carbohydrates: 14g
- Fiber: 3g
- Protein: 2g
- Sodium: 250mg

Creamy Butternut Squash Soup

Preparation Time: 10 minutes
Cooking Time: 30 minutes
Servings: 4

Ingredients:
- 1 medium peeled, seeded, and diced butternut squash
- 1 tablespoon olive oil
- 1 small onion, chopped
- 2 cloves garlic, minced
- 4 cups low-sodium vegetable broth
- 1 teaspoon ground cinnamon
- 1/2 teaspoon ground nutmeg
- Salt and pepper, to taste
- 1/2 cup low-fat coconut milk

- Fresh parsley or chives, for garnish (optional)

Directions:

1. In a big pot, heat olive oil over medium heat. Add chopped onion and garlic, and sauté until softened, about 5 minutes.
2. Add diced butternut squash to the pot and cook for another 5 minutes, stirring occasionally.
3. Pour in vegetable broth and season with ground cinnamon, ground nutmeg, salt, and pepper. Bring the mixture to a boil, then reduce the heat and let it simmer for 20 minutes or until the squash is tender.
4. Remove the pot from heat and let the mixture cool slightly.
5. Puree the soup until smooth and creamy using an immersion blender or regular blender,
6. Return the soup to the pot and stir in low-fat coconut milk. Heat the soup over low heat until warmed through.
7. Ladle the creamy butternut squash soup into individual containers for meal prep.
8. Garnish with fresh parsley or chives, if desired.
9. Store the prepared meal containers in the refrigerator for up to 4 days.

Nutrition Value (per serving):

- Calories: 160 kcal
- Fat: 5g
- Sodium: 200mg
- Carbohydrates: 30g
- Fiber: 5g
- Sugars: 7g
- Protein: 3g

Black Bean Soup

Preparation Time: 10 minutes
Cooking Time: 20 minutes
Servings: 4

Ingredients:

- 2 cans (15 oz each) drained and rinsed black beans
- 1 onion, chopped
- 2 cloves garlic, minced
- 1 red bell pepper, diced
- 1 can (14.5 oz) diced tomatoes
- 4 cups vegetable broth
- 1 teaspoon ground cumin
- 1 teaspoon chilli powder
- Salt and pepper to taste
- Fresh cilantro, chopped (for garnish)
- Lime wedges (for serving)

Directions:

1. In a large pot, sauté the chopped onion and garlic over medium heat until softened, about 5 minutes.
2. Add the diced red bell pepper to the pot and cook for another 3 minutes.
3. Stir in the drained and rinsed black beans, diced tomatoes, vegetable broth, ground cumin, and chilli powder. Season with salt and pepper to taste.
4. Bring the soup to a simmer and let it cook for about 15 minutes, allowing the flavours to meld together.
5. Once the soup is heated through and the vegetables are tender, remove it from the heat.
6. Use an immersion blender to partially blend the soup until it reaches your desired consistency. Alternatively, transfer half of the soup to a blender and blend until smooth, then return it to the pot.
7. Portion the black bean soup into meal prep containers, garnishing each serving with fresh cilantro. Place lime wedges in separate compartments or small containers for squeezing over the soup before eating.
8. Once cooled, seal the meal prep containers and refrigerate for up to 3-4 days.

Nutrition Value (per serving):

- Calories: 250
- Fat: 1.5g
- Sodium: 600mg
- Carbohydrates: 46g
- Dietary Fiber: 14g
- Sugars: 7g
- Protein: 14g

Spinach and White Bean Soup

Preparation Time: 10 minutes
Cooking Time: 20 minutes
Servings: 4

Ingredients:

- 1 tablespoon olive oil
- 1 onion, diced
- 2 cloves garlic, minced
- 4 cups low-sodium vegetable broth
- 2 cans (15 ounces each) white beans, drained and rinsed
- 4 cups fresh spinach leaves
- 1 teaspoon dried thyme
- Salt and pepper to taste
- Optional: freshly grated Parmesan cheese for serving

Directions:

1. In a big pot, heat olive oil over medium heat. Add diced onion and minced garlic, and cook until softened about 5 minutes.
2. Pour in vegetable broth and bring to a simmer.
3. Add white beans to the pot and simmer for 10 minutes to allow flavours to meld.
4. Stir in fresh spinach leaves and dried thyme, and cook until spinach is wilted about 5 minutes.
5. Season with pepper and salt to taste.
6. Ladle the soup into meal prep containers.
7. Optionally, sprinkle each serving with freshly grated Parmesan cheese.
8. Store the prepared soup in the refrigerator for up to 4 days.

Nutrition Value (per serving):
- Calories: 240
- Total Fat: 5g
- Sodium: 280mg
- Total Carbohydrates: 35g
- Dietary Fiber: 10g
- Sugars: 2g
- Protein: 13g

Broccoli Cheddar Soup

Preparation Time: 10 minutes
Cooking Time: 20 minutes
Servings: 4

Ingredients:
- 1 tablespoon olive oil
- 1 onion, chopped
- 2 cloves garlic, minced
- 4 cups chopped broccoli florets
- 3 cups low-sodium vegetable broth
- 1 cup low-fat milk
- 1 cup shredded cheddar cheese
- Salt and pepper, to taste
- Optional: ¼ teaspoon paprika

Directions:
1. Heat olive oil in a large pot over medium heat. Add chopped onion and minced garlic. Cook for 2-3 minutes until onion is soft and translucent.
2. Add chopped broccoli florets to the pot and cook for another 2-3 minutes, stirring occasionally.
3. Pour in the low-sodium vegetable broth and bring to a simmer. Let the soup simmer for about 10-15 minutes until the broccoli is tender.

4. Using an immersion blender or regular blender, blend the soup until smooth.

5. Return the soup to the pot over low heat. Stir in low-fat milk and shredded cheddar cheese until the cheese is melted and the soup is creamy.

6. Season with salt, pepper, and optional paprika, to taste. Adjust seasoning as needed.

7. Divide the soup into meal prep containers. Let cool completely before covering and storing in the refrigerator.

Nutrition Value per Serving (approx.):
- Calories: 220 kcal
- Protein: 12g
- Carbohydrates: 14g
- Fat: 14g
- Sodium: 350mg

Turkey and Vegetable Chilli Soup

Preparation time: 15 minutes
Cooking time: 25 minutes
Servings: 6

Ingredients:
- 1 tablespoon olive oil
- 1 onion, chopped

- 2 cloves garlic, minced
- 1 pound lean ground turkey
- 1 bell pepper, diced
- 1 zucchini, diced
- 1 can (15 ounces) diced tomatoes, undrained
- 1 can (15 ounces) kidney beans, drained and rinsed
- 1 can (15 ounces) black beans, drained and rinsed
- 2 cups low-sodium chicken broth
- 2 tablespoons chilli powder
- 1 teaspoon cumin
- 1/2 teaspoon paprika
- Salt and pepper, to taste

Directions:

1. Heat olive oil in a large pot over medium heat. Add the chopped onion and minced garlic, and cook until softened about 3 minutes.
2. Add the ground turkey to the pot and cook until browned, breaking it up with a spoon as it cooks, about 5 minutes.
3. Stir in the diced bell pepper and zucchini, and cook for another 3 minutes.
4. Add the diced tomatoes, kidney beans, black beans, chicken broth, chilli powder, cumin, paprika, salt, and pepper to the pot. Stir well to combine.

5. Bring the chilli to a simmer, then reduce the heat to low. Cover and let it simmer for 15 minutes, stirring occasionally.
6. After 15 minutes, taste and adjust seasoning if needed. Serve the chilli in meal prep containers, dividing evenly.
7. Let the chilli cool completely before covering and refrigerating or freezing for future meals.

Nutrition value per serving (1/6 of recipe):
- Calories: 290 kcal
- Protein: 23g
- Fat: 9g
- Carbohydrates: 28g
- Fiber: 8g
- Sodium: 390mg

Mushroom Barley Soup

Preparation Time: 10 minutes
Cooking Time: 30 minutes
Servings: 4

Ingredients:
- 1 tablespoon olive oil
- 1 onion, diced
- 2 cloves garlic, minced
- 8 ounces mushrooms, sliced

- 1 carrot, diced
- 1 celery stalk, diced
- 1/2 cup pearl barley, rinsed
- 4 cups vegetable broth (low-sodium)
- 2 cups water
- Salt and pepper to taste
- Fresh parsley, chopped (for garnish, optional)

Directions:

- Heat olive oil in a big pot over medium heat. Add diced onion and minced garlic. Cook until softened, about 5 minutes.
- Add sliced mushrooms, diced carrots, and diced celery to the pot. Cook until vegetables are tender, about 5 minutes.
- Stir in rinsed pearl barley and cook for 1 minute.
- Pour in vegetable broth and water. Bring the soup to a boil, then reduce heat to low and
- simmer, covered, for 25 minutes or until barley is tender.
- Season with salt and pepper to taste.
- Garnish with chopped parsley if desired.
- Divide the soup into meal prep containers. Let cool before refrigerating or freezing.

Nutrition Value (per serving):
- Calories: 200

- Protein: 5g
- Fat: 4g
- Carbohydrates: 35g
- Fiber: 6g
- Sodium: 250mg

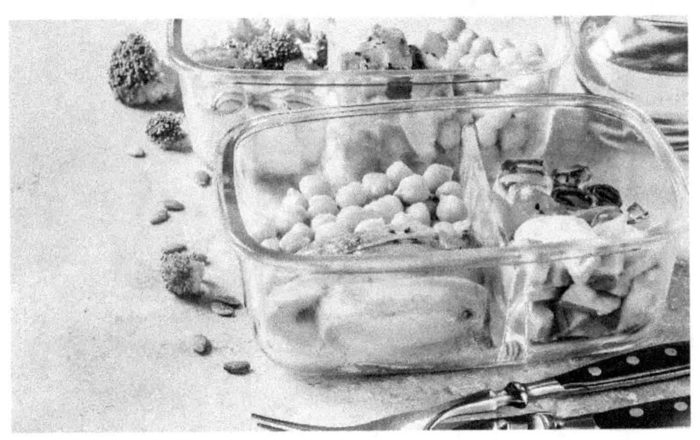

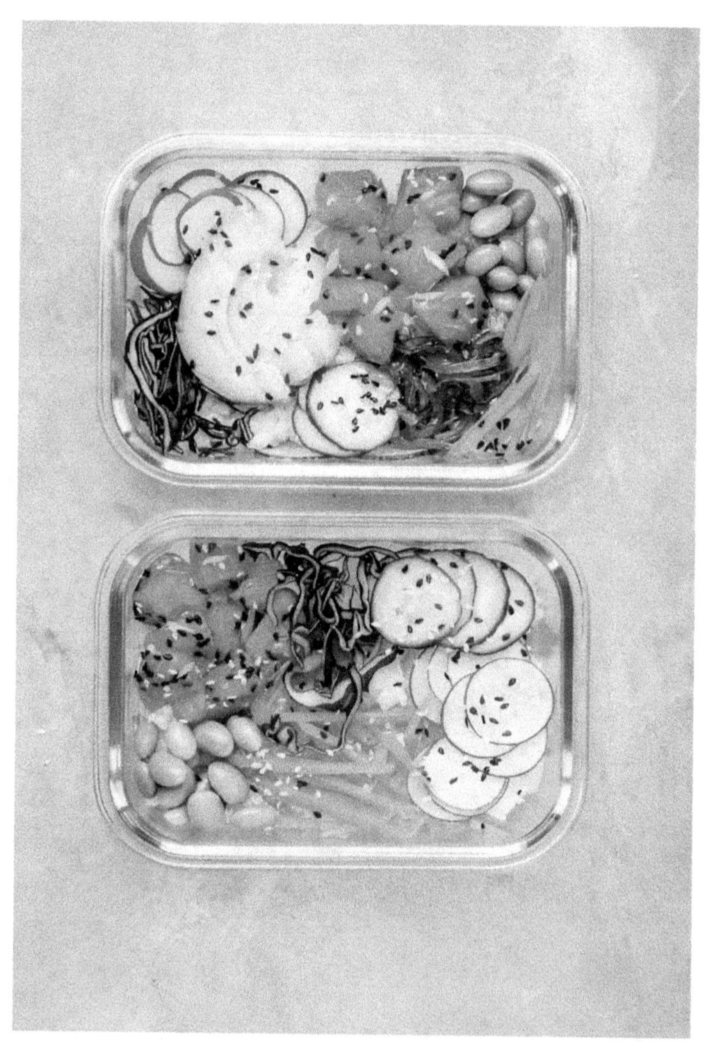

Chapter 6: Snack Attack

Fruit Salad with Mint and Lime

Preparation time: 10 minutes
Servings: 4

Ingredients:
- 2 cups mixed fruits (such as strawberries, blueberries, grapes, and pineapple), chopped
- 2 tablespoons fresh mint leaves, chopped
- 1 lime, juiced

Directions:
- In a large bowl, combine the mixed fruits and chopped mint leaves.
- Squeeze the juice of one lime over the fruit mixture.
- Gently toss the fruit salad until everything is evenly coated with lime juice.
- Divide the fruit salad into individual airtight containers.
- Seal the containers and store them in the refrigerator for up to 3-4 days.

Nutrition Value (per serving):
- Calories: 45 kcal
- Protein: 0.5g
- Carbohydrates: 11g

- Fat: 0.2g
- Fiber: 2g
- Sugar: 7g
- Sodium: 1mg

Hummus and Pita Bread

Preparation time: 10 minutes
Cooking time: 5 minutes
Servings: 4

Ingredients:
- 1 can (15 ounces) chickpeas, drained and rinsed
- 2 cloves garlic, minced
- 1/4 cup tahini
- 2 tablespoons lemon juice
- 2 tablespoons olive oil
- Salt to taste
- 4 whole wheat pita bread rounds

Directions:
1. In a food processor or blender, combine the chickpeas, minced garlic, tahini, lemon juice, olive oil, and salt.
2. Blend until smooth and creamy, adding a little water if necessary to reach your desired consistency.

3. Divide the hummus into individual airtight containers.
4. Cut the whole wheat pita bread into wedges.
5. Store the pita bread wedges in a separate airtight container.
6. Keep both containers refrigerated for up to 4-5 days.

Nutrition Value (per serving - 2 tablespoons of hummus with 1 whole wheat pita bread round):
- Calories: 240 kcal
- Protein: 8g
- Carbohydrates: 32g
- Fat: 10g
- Fiber: 6g
- Sugar: 1g
- Sodium: 380mg

Greek Yoghurt with Honey and Almonds

Preparation time: 5 minutes
Servings: 1

Ingredients:
- 1/2 cup Greek yogurt
- 1 tablespoon honey
- 1 tablespoon sliced almonds

Directions:

- In a bowl, spoon Greek yoghurt.
- Drizzle honey over the yoghurt.
- Sprinkle sliced almonds on top.
- Stir gently to combine.
- Seal the container and store it in the refrigerator for up to 3-4 days.

Nutrition Value (per serving):

- Calories: 180 kcal
- Protein: 12g
- Carbohydrates: 17g
- Fat: 8g
- Fiber: 2g
- Sugar: 15g
- Sodium: 50mg

Ants on a Log (Celery with Peanut Butter and Raisins)

Preparation time: 5 minutes
Cooking time: 0 minutes
Servings: 2

Ingredients:

- 4 celery stalks
- 2 tablespoons peanut butter
- 2 tablespoons raisins

Directions:

1. Wash and dry the celery stalks, then cut them into halves or thirds, depending on your preference.
2. Spread peanut butter onto each celery piece using a butter knife.
3. Press raisins into the peanut butter along the length of each celery piece.
4. Place the prepared Ants on a Log in an airtight container or on a plate covered with plastic wrap.
5. Store in the refrigerator until ready to eat.

Nutrition Value (per serving):

- Calories: 150 kcal
- Protein: 4g
- Carbohydrates: 15g
- Fat: 9g
- Fiber: 3g
- Sugar: 9g
- Sodium: 110mg

Edamame with Sea Salt

Preparation time: 5 minutes
Cooking time: 5 minutes
Servings: 2

Ingredients:
- 2 cups frozen edamame (shelled)
- 1 tablespoon sea salt

Directions:
1. Bring a pot of water to a boil on high heat.
2. Add the frozen edamame to the boiling water and cook for 5 minutes.
3. The edamame should be drained and transferred to a bowl.
4. Sprinkle the cooked edamame with sea salt and toss to coat evenly.
5. Allow the edamame to cool completely before storing them in an airtight container in the refrigerator.

Nutrition Value (per serving):
- Calories: 120 kcal
- Protein: 11g
- Carbohydrates: 9g
- Fat: 4g
- Fiber: 5g
- Sugar: 2g
- Sodium: 1170mg

Popcorn with Olive Oil and Parmesan Cheese

Preparation time: 5 minutes
Cooking time: 5 minutes
Servings: 2

Ingredients:
- 1/2 cup popcorn kernels
- 2 tablespoons olive oil
- 1/4 cup grated Parmesan cheese
- Salt to taste

Directions:
1. Heat the olive oil in a big pot over medium heat.
2. Add the popcorn kernels to the pot and cover with a lid.
3. Cook the popcorn, shaking the pot occasionally, until the popping sound slows down, about 3-5 minutes.
4. Remove the pot from heat and let it sit for a minute to allow any remaining kernels to pop.
5. Transfer the popped popcorn to a large bowl.
6. Drizzle the popcorn with olive oil and sprinkle with grated Parmesan cheese.

7. Add salt to taste and toss the popcorn until evenly coated.

8. Allow the popcorn to cool completely before storing it in an airtight container in the pantry.

Nutrition Value (per serving):
- Calories: 250 kcal
- Protein: 5g
- Carbohydrates: 18g
- Fat: 18g
- Fiber: 4g
- Sugar: 0g
- Sodium: 200mg

Cucumber Slices with Cream Cheese and Dill

Preparation time: 5 minutes
Servings: 2

Ingredients:
- 1 large cucumber
- 4 tablespoons cream cheese
- Fresh dill, for garnish

Directions:

1. Wash the cucumber and slice it into thin rounds.
2. Spread a thin layer of cream cheese onto each cucumber slice.
3. Garnish with fresh dill on top of the cream cheese.
4. Arrange the prepared cucumber slices in an airtight container.
5. Seal the container and store it in the refrigerator until ready to eat.

Nutrition Value (per serving):

- Calories: 70 kcal
- Protein: 2g
- Carbohydrates: 4g
- Fat: 5g
- Fiber: 1g
- Sugar: 2g
- Sodium: 80mg

Almond Butter and Banana Rice Cakes

Preparation time: 5 minutes
Cooking time: 0 minutes
Servings: 1

Ingredients:

- 2 rice cakes

- 2 tablespoons almond butter
- 1 ripe banana, sliced
- Optional toppings: honey, cinnamon

Directions:

1. Spread 1 tablespoon of almond butter onto each rice cake.
2. Top each rice cake with slices of banana.
3. Drizzle with honey and sprinkle with cinnamon, if desired.
4. Store the prepared rice cakes in an airtight container in the refrigerator.

Nutrition Value (per serving):

- Calories: 340 kcal
- Protein: 7g
- Carbohydrates: 46g
- Fat: 16g
- Fiber: 5g
- Sugar: 17g
- Sodium: 60mg

Trail Mix with Dried Fruit and Nuts

Preparation time: 5 minutes
Servings: 4

Ingredients:

- 1 cup mixed nuts (almonds, walnuts, and cashews)
- 1/2 cup dried fruit (such as raisins, cranberries, and apricots)
- 1/4 cup dark chocolate chips (optional)

Directions:

1. In a large bowl, combine the mixed nuts, dried fruit, and dark chocolate chips, if using.
2. Gently toss the ingredients together until evenly distributed.
3. Divide the trail mix into 4 equal portions.
4. Transfer each portion into a small zip-top bag or airtight container.
5. Seal the bags or containers and store them in a cool, dry place until ready to enjoy.

Nutrition Value (per serving):

- Calories: 200 kcal
- Protein: 5g
- Carbohydrates: 20g
- Fat: 12g
- Fiber: 3g
- Sugar: 14g
- Sodium: 5mg

Greek Yogurt Dip with Sliced Vegetables

Preparation time: 5 minutes
Cooking time: 0 minutes
Servings: 4

Ingredients:

- 1 cup Greek yogurt
- 1 tablespoon lemon juice
- 1 teaspoon chopped dried dill or 1 tablespoon fresh dill
- 1/2 teaspoon garlic powder
- Salt and pepper to taste
- Assorted sliced vegetables (such as carrots, cucumbers, bell peppers, and cherry tomatoes)

Directions:

1. In a mixing bowl, combine the Greek yoghurt, lemon juice, dried dill, garlic powder, salt, and pepper. Stir until well combined.
2. Transfer the yoghurt dip to an airtight container.
3. Wash and slice the assorted vegetables into bite-sized pieces.
4. Store the sliced vegetables in a separate container.
5. Keep both containers in the refrigerator until ready to serve.

Nutrition Value (per serving, dip only):
- Calories: 30 kcal
- Protein: 6g
- Carbohydrates: 2g
- Fat: 0g
- Fiber: 0g
- Sugar: 2g
- Sodium: 20mg

Baked Sweet Potato Fries with Spicy Ketchup

Preparation time: 10 minutes
Cooking time: 25 minutes
Servings: 2

Ingredients:

- 2 medium peeled sweet potatoes and cut into fries
- 1 tablespoon olive oil
- Salt and pepper to taste
- 1/4 cup ketchup
- 1/2 teaspoon hot sauce (adjust to taste)

Directions:

1. Preheat the oven to 425°F (220°C). Line a baking sheet with parchment paper.
2. In a large bowl, toss the sweet potato fries with olive oil, salt, and pepper until evenly coated.
3. Spread the fries in a single layer on the prepared baking sheet, making sure they are not overcrowded.
4. Bake for 20-25 minutes, flipping halfway through, until the fries are golden brown and crispy.
5. While the fries are baking, mix together the ketchup and hot sauce in a small bowl to make the spicy ketchup.
6. Once the fries are done, remove them from the oven and allow them to cool completely.
7. Divide the fries into meal prep containers and store them in the refrigerator.

8. Pour the spicy ketchup into small containers or portion them out into individual servings.

9. When ready to eat, reheat the sweet potato fries in the microwave until warmed through.

10. Serve with the spicy ketchup for dipping.

Nutrition Value (per serving):
- Calories: 200 kcal
- Protein: 2g
- Carbohydrates: 35g
- Fat: 6g
- Fiber: 5g
- Sugar: 10g
- Sodium: 420mg

Cherry Tomatoes with Mozzarella Balls and Basil

Preparation time: 5 minutes
Cooking time: 0 minutes
Servings: 2

Ingredients:
- 1 cup cherry tomatoes
- 1/2 cup mini mozzarella balls
- Fresh basil leaves, torn
- 1 tablespoon balsamic glaze (optional)
- Salt and pepper to taste

Directions:

1. Rinse the cherry tomatoes and pat them dry with a paper towel.
2. In a small bowl, combine the cherry tomatoes and mini mozzarella balls.
3. Tear fresh basil leaves and sprinkle them over the tomatoes and mozzarella.
4. Season with pepper and salt to taste.
5. Drizzle with balsamic glaze if desired.
6. Gently toss everything together until evenly combined.
7. Divide the mixture into meal prep containers.
8. Seal the containers and store them in the refrigerator for up to 3 days.

Nutrition Value (per serving):

- Calories: 120 kcal
- Protein: 6g
- Carbohydrates: 4g
- Fat: 9g
- Fiber: 1g
- Sugar: 2g
- Sodium: 200mg

Apple Slices with Cinnamon and Almond Butter

Preparation time: 5 minutes
Servings: 1

Ingredients:
- 1 medium apple, sliced
- 1 tablespoon almond butter
- 1/4 teaspoon ground cinnamon

Directions:
1. Slice the apple into thin slices.
2. In a small bowl, mix the almond butter with ground cinnamon until well combined.
3. Place the apple slices in an airtight container.
4. Pack the cinnamon almond butter in a separate small container.
5. Store both containers in the refrigerator until ready to eat.

Nutrition Value (per serving):
- Calories: 150 kcal
- Protein: 3g
- Carbohydrates: 19g
- Fat: 8g
- Fiber: 5g
- Sugar: 14g

- Sodium: 0mg

Homemade Guacamole with Baked Tortilla Chips

Preparation time: 10 minutes
Cooking time: 10 minutes
Servings: 4

Ingredients:
- 2 ripe avocados
- 1 small tomato, diced
- 1/4 cup red onion, finely chopped
- 1 clove garlic, minced
- 1 tablespoon lime juice
- Salt and pepper to taste
- 4 small corn tortillas

Directions:
1. Preheat your oven to 350°F (175°C).
2. Cut the corn tortillas into wedges and place them in a single layer on a baking sheet lined with parchment paper.
3. Bake the tortilla chips in the preheated oven for 8-10 minutes, or until crispy and golden brown. Remove from the oven and allow them to cool completely before storing.
4. While the tortilla chips are baking, prepare the guacamole. Cut the avocados in half,

remove the pits, and scoop the flesh into a mixing bowl.

5. Mash the avocado with a fork until smooth or leave it slightly chunky if desired.

6. Add the diced tomato, chopped red onion, minced garlic, lime juice, salt, and pepper to the mashed avocado. Stir until well combined.

7. Transfer the guacamole to an airtight container and store it in the refrigerator until ready to eat.

Nutrition Value (per serving, including 1/4 of guacamole and tortilla chips):
- Calories: 180 kcal
- Protein: 3g
- Carbohydrates: 20g
- Fat: 11g
- Fiber: 7g
- Sugar: 2g
- Sodium: 70mg

Stuffed Dates with Cream Cheese and Pistachios

Preparation time: 10 minutes
Cooking time: 0 minutes
Servings: 12

Ingredients:
- 12 Medjool dates, pitted
- 2 ounces cream cheese, softened
- 1/4 cup shelled pistachios, chopped

Directions:
1. Using a small knife, make a lengthwise slit in each date and remove the pit.
2. In a small bowl, mix the softened cream cheese and chopped pistachios until well combined.
3. Gently stuff each date with a spoonful of the cream cheese mixture, pressing lightly to close the opening.
4. Place the stuffed dates in an airtight container, separating layers with parchment paper if needed.
5. Store in the refrigerator for up to 5 days.

Nutrition Value (per serving - 1 stuffed date):
- Calories: 80 kcal
- Protein: 1g
- Carbohydrates: 14g
- Fat: 3g
- Fiber: 1g
- Sugar: 12g
- Sodium: 15mg

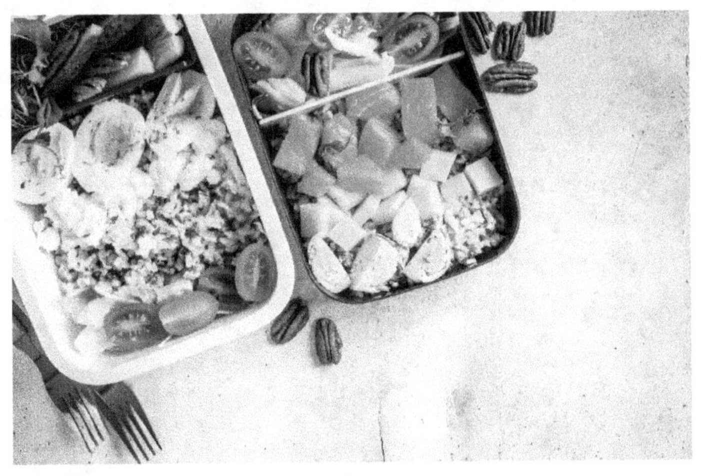

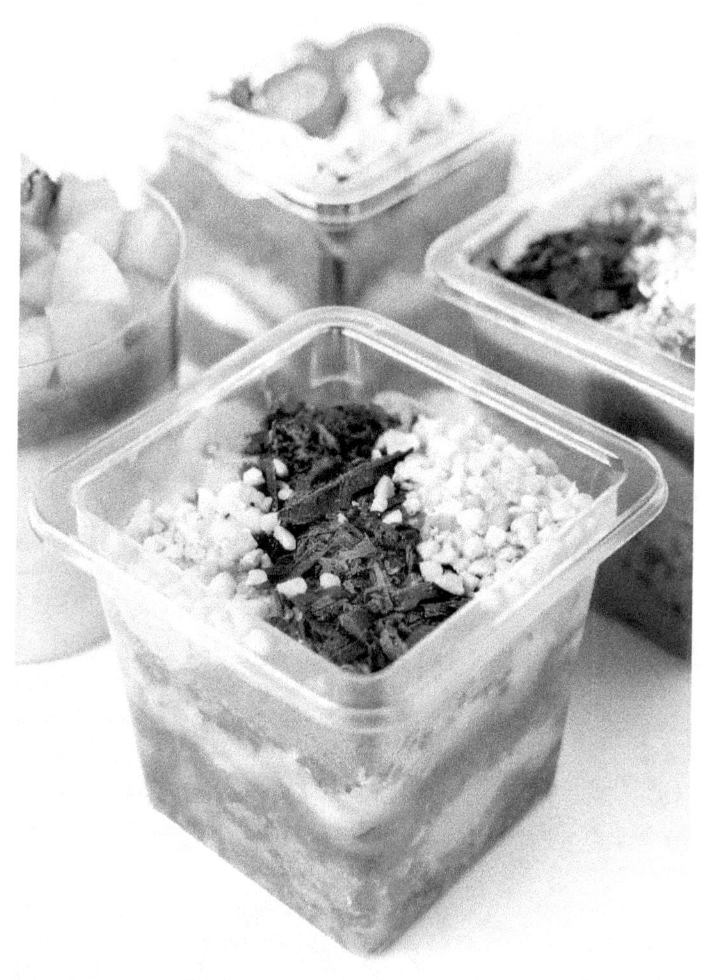

Chapter 7: Sweet Treats and Desserts

Berry Smoothie Bowl with Granola and Coconut Flakes

Preparation time: 5 minutes
Servings: 1

Ingredients:
- 1 cup mixed berries (strawberries, blueberries, raspberries)
- 1/2 ripe banana
- 1/2 cup Greek yogurt
- 1/4 cup almond milk
- 1/4 cup granola
- 2 tablespoons coconut flakes

Directions:
1. In a blender, combine the mixed berries, banana, Greek yoghurt, and almond milk.
2. Blend until smooth and creamy.
3. Pour the smoothie into a bowl.
4. Top with granola and coconut flakes.
5. Seal the bowl with an airtight lid and store it in the refrigerator for up to 2 days.

Nutrition Value (per serving):

- Calories: 350 kcal
- Protein: 15g
- Carbohydrates: 45g
- Fat: 13g
- Fiber: 8g
- Sugar: 22g
- Sodium: 80mg

Chocolate Avocado Mousse with Fresh Berries

Preparation time: 10 minutes
Servings: 2

Ingredients:
- 1 ripe avocado
- 2 tablespoons cocoa powder
- 2 tablespoons honey or maple syrup
- 1 teaspoon vanilla extract
- 1/4 cup almond milk (or any milk of your choice)
- Fresh berries for topping (such as strawberries, blueberries, raspberries)

Directions:

1. Halve the avocado, remove the pit, and transfer the flesh to a food processor or blender.
2. Add the cocoa powder, honey or maple syrup, vanilla extract, and almond milk to the blender.
3. Blend until smooth and creamy, scraping down the sides as needed.
4. Divide the mousse into two small containers or jars with lids.
5. Seal the containers and store them in the refrigerator for up to 3-4 days.
6. When ready to eat, top each serving with fresh berries before serving.

Nutrition Value (per serving):

- Calories: 200 kcal
- Protein: 3g
- Carbohydrates: 25g
- Fat: 12g
- Fiber: 7g
- Sugar: 15g
- Sodium: 10mg

Baked Cinnamon Apple Slices with Greek Yogurt

Preparation time: 10 minutes
Cooking time: 20 minutes
Servings: 2

Ingredients:
- 2 apples, cored and thinly sliced
- 1 tablespoon honey
- 1 teaspoon ground cinnamon
- 1 cup Greek yogurt
- Optional toppings: chopped nuts, granola

Directions:
1. Preheat your oven to 375°F (190°C).
2. In a mixing bowl, toss the apple slices with honey and cinnamon until evenly coated.
3. Spread the apple slices in a single layer on a baking sheet lined with parchment paper.
4. Bake in the preheated oven for 15-20 minutes, or until the apples are tender and lightly caramelized.
5. Allow the baked apple slices to cool completely before transferring them to an airtight container.
6. Divide the Greek yoghurt into two separate containers.

7. When ready to eat, serve the baked apple slices with Greek yoghurt and any desired optional toppings.

Nutrition Value (per serving):
- Calories: 180 kcal
- Protein: 10g
- Carbohydrates: 35g
- Fat: 1g
- Fiber: 5g
- Sugar: 25g
- Sodium: 60mg

Pistachio Date Balls with Coconut

Preparation time: 15 minutes
Cooking time: 0 minutes
Servings: 12 balls

Ingredients:
- 1 cup pitted dates
- 1/2 cup shelled pistachios
- 1/4 cup shredded coconut
- 1 tablespoon honey
- 1/2 teaspoon vanilla extract
- Pinch of salt

Directions:

1. Place the dates and pistachios in a food processor and pulse until finely chopped and combined.
2. Add the shredded coconut, honey, vanilla extract, and salt to the food processor. Pulse until the mixture comes together and forms a sticky dough.
3. Scoop out tablespoon-sized portions of the mixture and roll into balls using your hands.
4. Place the balls onto a parchment paper-lined baking sheet.
5. Optional: Roll the balls in additional shredded coconut for extra coating.
6. Store the Pistachio Date Balls with Coconut in an airtight container in the refrigerator for up to one week.

Nutrition Value (per serving - 1 ball):
- Calories: 80 kcal
- Protein: 1g
- Carbohydrates: 14g
- Fat: 3g
- Fiber: 2g
- Sugar: 11g
- Sodium: 5mg

Pineapple Banana Ice Cream

Preparation time: 5 minutes
Freezing time: 3 hours
Servings: 2

Ingredients:
- 2 ripe bananas, sliced and frozen
- 1 cup frozen pineapple chunks

Directions:
1. Place the frozen banana slices and frozen pineapple chunks in a blender or food processor.
2. Blend while scraping down the sides as needed until smooth and creamy.
3. Transfer the mixture to a shallow dish or container and spread it out evenly.
4. Cover the dish or container with a lid or plastic wrap.
5. Place in the freezer for at least 3 hours, or until firm.
6. Once frozen, scoop the pineapple banana ice cream into airtight containers.
7. Store containers in the freezer.

Nutrition Value (per serving):
- Calories: 110 kcal
- Protein: 1g
- Carbohydrates: 28g

- Fat: 0g
- Fiber: 3g
- Sugar: 16g
- Sodium: 1mg

Dark Chocolate Covered Almonds

Preparation time: 5 minutes
Cooking time: 5 minutes
Servings: 4

Ingredients:
- 1 cup raw almonds
- 4 ounces dark chocolate (at least 70% cocoa)

Directions:
1. Line a baking sheet a silicone baking mat or a parchment paper.
2. In a microwave-safe bowl, melt the dark chocolate in 30-second intervals, stirring in between, until smooth and fully melted.
3. Add the raw almonds to the melted chocolate and stir until all the almonds are evenly coated.
4. Use a fork or a slotted spoon to transfer the chocolate-covered almonds to the prepared baking sheet, arranging them in a single layer.

5. Place the baking sheet in the refrigerator for 30 minutes, or until the chocolate has set.
6. Once the chocolate has hardened, transfer the chocolate-covered almonds to an airtight container or zip-top bag for storage.
7. Store the chocolate-covered almonds in the refrigerator for up to 2 weeks.

Nutrition Value (per serving - about 1/4 cup):
- Calories: 200 kcal
- Protein: 5g
- Carbohydrates: 10g
- Fat: 15g
- Fiber: 3g
- Sugar: 5g
- Sodium: 0mg

Strawberry Yogurt Bark with Pistachios

Preparation time: 10 minutes
Freezing time: 3 hours
Servings: 4

Ingredients:
- 2 cups plain Greek yoghurt
- 1 cup fresh strawberries, sliced
- 1/4 cup pistachios, chopped
- 2 tablespoons honey

Directions:

1. Line a baking sheet with parchment paper.
2. In a bowl, mix Greek yoghurt and honey until well combined.
3. Spread the yoghurt mixture evenly onto the prepared baking sheet.
4. Distribute sliced strawberries and chopped pistachios over the yoghurt.
5. Place the baking sheet in the freezer and let it freeze for at least 3 hours or until firm.
6. Once frozen, break the yoghurt bark into pieces.
7. Store the pieces in an airtight container in the freezer until ready to serve.

Nutrition Value (per serving):
- Calories: 120 kcal
- Protein: 10g
- Carbohydrates: 14g
- Fat: 4g
- Fiber: 2g
- Sugar: 10g
- Sodium: 25mg

Coconut Macaroons with Chocolate Drizzle

Preparation time: 10 minutes

Cooking time: 15 minutes
Servings: 12

Ingredients:
- 2 cups unsweetened shredded coconut
- 1/2 cup sweetened condensed milk
- 1 teaspoon vanilla extract
- 2 large egg whites
- 1/4 teaspoon salt
- 1/2 cup dark chocolate chips

Directions:
1. Preheat the oven to 325°F (160°C) and line a baking sheet with parchment paper.
2. Combine the shredded coconut, sweetened condensed milk, and vanilla extract in a large bowl and mix well.
3. Beat the egg whites and salt in a separate bowl until stiff peaks form.
4. Gently fold the beaten egg whites into the coconut mixture until fully combined.
5. Using a spoon or cookie scoop, drop rounded tablespoons of the mixture onto the prepared baking sheet, spacing them about 1 inch apart.
6. Bake for 12-15 minutes, or until the macaroons are golden brown around the edges.

7. Allow the macaroons to cool completely on the baking sheet.
8. In a microwave-safe bowl, melt the dark chocolate chips in 30-second intervals, stirring until smooth.
9. Drizzle the melted chocolate over the cooled macaroons.
10. Allow the chocolate to set before storing the macaroons in an airtight container in the refrigerator.

Nutrition Value (per serving):
- Calories: 160 kcal
- Protein: 2g
- Carbohydrates: 13g
- Fat: 11g
- Fiber: 2g
- Sugar: 10g
- Sodium: 85mg

Raspberry Oatmeal Bars

Preparation time: 10 minutes
Cooking time: 30 minutes
Servings: 12 bars

Ingredients:
- 2 cups old-fashioned oats
- 1 cup whole wheat flour

- 1/2 cup packed brown sugar
- 1 teaspoon baking powder
- 1/4 teaspoon salt
- 1/2 cup unsweetened applesauce
- 1/4 cup honey
- 1/4 cup melted coconut oil
- 1 teaspoon vanilla extract
- 1 cup fresh raspberries

Directions:

1. Preheat your oven to 350°F (175°C) and grease a 9x9-inch baking dish.
2. In a large bowl, mix together the oats, flour, brown sugar, baking powder, and salt.
3. Add the applesauce, honey, melted coconut oil, and vanilla extract to the dry ingredients. Mix until well combined.
4. Press two-thirds of the oat mixture into the bottom of the prepared baking dish, forming an even layer.
5. Scatter the fresh raspberries evenly over the oat layer.
6. Sprinkle the remaining oat mixture over the raspberries, pressing down gently.
7. Bake in the preheated oven for 25-30 minutes, or until the top is golden brown.
8. Allow the bars to cool completely in the baking dish before cutting them into squares.

9. Store the raspberry oatmeal bars in an airtight container in the refrigerator for up to 5 days.

Nutrition Value (per serving):
- Calories: 180 kcal
- Protein: 3g
- Carbohydrates: 29g
- Fat: 6g
- Fiber: 3g
- Sugar: 12g
- Sodium: 60mg

Vanilla Bean Rice Pudding with Cinnamon

Preparation time: 5 minutes
Cooking time: 25 minutes
Servings: 4

Ingredients:
- 1 cup uncooked white rice
- 2 cups unsweetened almond milk
- 1/4 cup maple syrup
- 1 vanilla bean, split and seeds scraped out (or 1 teaspoon vanilla extract)
- 1/2 teaspoon ground cinnamon
- Pinch of salt

- Optional toppings: additional cinnamon, sliced almonds, fresh fruit

Directions:
1. In a medium saucepan, combine the uncooked white rice, almond milk, maple syrup, vanilla bean seeds (or vanilla extract), ground cinnamon, and a pinch of salt.
2. Bring the mixture to a boil over medium heat, then reduce the heat to low and simmer uncovered, stirring occasionally, for 20-25 minutes or until the rice is tender and the pudding has thickened to your desired consistency.
3. Remove the saucepan from the heat and let the rice pudding cool slightly.
4. Divide the rice pudding evenly into meal prep containers.
5. Allow the rice pudding to cool completely before sealing the containers and storing them in the refrigerator for up to 3-4 days.

Nutrition Value (per serving):
- Calories: 220 kcal
- Protein: 3g
- Carbohydrates: 47g
- Fat: 2g
- Fiber: 1g
- Sugar: 15g

- Sodium: 100mg

Lemon Poppy Seed Muffins

Preparation time: 10 minutes
Cooking time: 20 minutes
Servings: 12 muffins

Ingredients:
- 2 cups all-purpose flour
- 3/4 cup sugar
- 2 teaspoons baking powder
- 1/2 teaspoon baking soda
- 1/4 teaspoon salt
- 1 cup Greek yogurt
- 1/4 cup olive oil
- 2 large eggs
- Zest of 2 lemons
- Juice of 1 lemon
- 2 tablespoons poppy seeds

Directions:

1. Preheat the oven to 375°F (190°C). Lightly grease with cooking spray or line a muffin tin with paper liners.
2. In a large mixing bowl, combine the flour, sugar, baking powder, baking soda, and salt.
3. In a separate bowl, whisk together the Greek yoghurt, olive oil, eggs, lemon zest, and lemon juice until smooth.
4. Mix the wet ingredients together with the dry ingredients and stir until just combined. Be careful not to overmix.
5. Gently fold in the poppy seeds until evenly distributed throughout the batter.
6. Spoon the batter into the prepared muffin tin, filling each cup about 3/4 full.
7. Bake for 18-20 minutes, or until the muffins are golden brown and a toothpick inserted into the centre comes out clean.
8. Allow the muffins to cool in the tin for 5 minutes, then transfer them to a wire rack to cool completely before storing.

Nutrition Value (per serving - 1 muffin):

- Calories: 200 kcal
- Protein: 5g
- Carbohydrates: 28g
- Fat: 8g
- Fiber: 1g

- Sugar: 13g
- Sodium: 180mg

Peanut Butter Energy Balls with Rolled Oats and Honey

Preparation time: 10 minutes
Servings: Makes about 12 balls

Ingredients:
- 1 cup rolled oats
- 1/2 cup peanut butter
- 1/4 cup honey
- 1/4 cup mini chocolate chips (optional)
- 1 teaspoon vanilla extract
- Pinch of salt

Directions:
1. Combine all ingredients in a mixing bowl.
2. Stir until well combined and the mixture holds together.
3. Roll the mixture into balls, about 1 inch in diameter, using your hands.
4. Transfer the balls to a parchment paper-lined baking sheet.
5. Refrigerate for at least 30 minutes to firm up.

6. Once firm, transfer the energy balls to an airtight container and store them in the refrigerator for up to one week.

Nutrition Value (per serving - 1 ball):
- Calories: 110 kcal
- Protein: 3g
- Carbohydrates: 11g
- Fat: 6g
- Fiber: 1g
- Sugar: 5g
- Sodium: 45mg

Orange Creamsicle Smoothie with Greek Yogurt

Preparation time: 5 minutes
Servings: 2

Ingredients:
- 1 cup Greek yoghurt
- 1 cup orange juice (freshly squeezed or store-bought)
- 1 ripe banana
- 1 teaspoon vanilla extract
- 1 tablespoon honey (optional)
- 1 cup ice cubes

Directions:

1. In a blender, combine Greek yoghurt, orange juice, banana, vanilla extract, and honey (if using).
2. Add ice cubes to the blender.
3. Blend on high speed until smooth and creamy, about 1-2 minutes.
4. Divide the smoothie between two glasses.
5. Serve immediately or store in airtight containers in the refrigerator for up to 24 hours.

Nutrition Value (per serving):
- Calories: 150 kcal
- Protein: 10g
- Carbohydrates: 30g
- Fat: 0g
- Fiber: 2g
- Sugar: 22g
- Sodium: 60mg

Baked Cinnamon Sugar Pita Chips with Fruit Salsa

Preparation time: 10 minutes
Cooking time: 10 minutes
Servings: 4

Ingredients:
- 4 whole wheat pita bread rounds

- 2 tablespoons olive oil
- 2 tablespoons granulated sugar
- 1 teaspoon ground cinnamon
- 2 cups mixed fresh fruit (such as strawberries, kiwi, pineapple, and mango), diced
- 1 tablespoon fresh lime juice
- 1 tablespoon honey

Directions:

1. Preheat the oven to 350°F (175°C).
2. Cut each pita bread round into 8 wedges.
3. In a small bowl, mix together the olive oil, granulated sugar, and ground cinnamon.
4. Brush both sides of the pita wedges with the cinnamon sugar mixture.
5. Place the pita wedges in a single layer on a baking sheet lined with parchment paper.
6. Bake for 8-10 minutes, or until the pita chips are golden brown and crispy.
7. While the pita chips are baking, prepare the fruit salsa by combining the diced mixed fruit, lime juice, and honey in a bowl. Mix well to coat the fruit evenly.
8. Remove the pita chips from the oven and allow them to cool completely.
9. Divide the baked cinnamon sugar pita chips into meal prep containers. Place the fruit

salsa in separate compartments or small containers for dipping.

10. Once cooled, seal the meal prep containers and refrigerate for up to 3-4 days.

Nutrition Value (per serving):
- Calories: 210 kcal
- Protein: 3g
- Carbohydrates: 36g
- Fat: 6g
- Fiber: 4g
- Sugar: 16g
- Sodium: 140mg

Chapter 8: DASH Diet For Special Occasions

Grilled Steak with Roasted Vegetables and Chimichurri Sauce

Preparation time: 15 minutes
Cooking time: 20 minutes
Servings: 2

Ingredients:

- 2 sirloin steaks, 8 ounces each
- Salt and pepper to taste
- 2 cups chopped mixed vegetables (bell peppers, zucchini, and red onion)
- 1 tablespoon olive oil
- 1/4 cup fresh parsley, chopped
- 2 tablespoons fresh cilantro, chopped
- 2 cloves garlic, minced
- 2 tablespoons red wine vinegar
- 1/4 cup olive oil
- 1/4 teaspoon red pepper flakes (optional)

Directions:

1. Preheat the grill to medium-high heat.
2. Season the steaks on both sides with pepper and salt.

3. In a bowl, toss the mixed vegetables with 1 tablespoon of olive oil and season with salt and pepper.
4. Grill the steaks for 3-4 minutes per side for medium-rare, or to your desired level of doneness. Remove the steak from the grill and let it rest for 5 minutes before slicing.
5. While the steaks are resting, grill the vegetables in a grill basket or on a sheet of aluminum foil for 8-10 minutes, or until tender and slightly charred.
6. In a small bowl, combine the chopped parsley, cilantro, minced garlic, red wine vinegar, olive oil, and red pepper flakes (if using) to make the chimichurri sauce.
7. Serve the sliced steak with the grilled vegetables and drizzle with chimichurri sauce.
8. Allow to cool completely before storing them in separate airtight containers in the refrigerator.

Nutrition Value (per serving):
- Calories: 450 kcal
- Protein: 30g
- Carbohydrates: 10g
- Fat: 32g
- Fiber: 3g
- Sugar: 3g

- Sodium: 80mg

Baked Chicken Alfredo with Whole Wheat Pasta

Preparation time: 15 minutes
Cooking time: 30 minutes
Servings: 4

Ingredients:
- 8 ounces whole wheat pasta
- 2 boneless, skinless chicken breasts, diced
- 2 cups broccoli florets
- 1 tablespoon olive oil
- 2 cloves garlic, minced
- 1 cup low-fat milk
- 1/2 cup grated Parmesan cheese
- Salt and pepper to taste

Directions:
1. Preheat your oven to 375°F (190°C). Cook the whole wheat pasta according to package instructions. Drain and set aside.
2. In a large skillet, heat the olive oil over medium heat. Add the diced chicken and cook until browned and cooked through about 5-6 minutes.
3. Add the minced garlic and broccoli florets to the skillet with the chicken. Cook for an

additional 2-3 minutes, until the broccoli is tender.

4. Pour in the low-fat milk and grated Parmesan cheese. Until the cheese has melted and the sauce is smooth, thoroughly stir. Season with pepper and salt to taste.
5. Add the cooked pasta to the skillet and toss until evenly coated with the sauce.
6. Transfer the chicken Alfredo mixture to a baking dish and spread it out evenly.
7. Bake in the preheated oven for 15-20 minutes, until the top is golden brown and bubbly.
8. Remove from the oven and let it cool completely before portioning it into meal prep containers.

Nutrition Value (per serving):
- Calories: 380 kcal
- Protein: 30g
- Carbohydrates: 35g
- Fat: 12g
- Fiber: 5g
- Sugar: 4g
- Sodium: 380mg

Shrimp Scampi with Zucchini Noodles

Preparation time: 10 minutes

Cooking time: 10 minutes
Servings: 2

Ingredients:
- 2 medium zucchini, spiralized into noodles
- 8 ounces medium shrimp, peeled and deveined
- 2 tablespoons olive oil
- 3 cloves garlic, minced
- 1/4 teaspoon red pepper flakes (optional)
- Salt and pepper to taste
- 1 tablespoon lemon juice
- 2 tablespoons chopped fresh parsley

Directions:
1. Heat 1 tablespoon of olive oil in a large skillet over medium heat.
2. Add the minced garlic and red pepper flakes (if using) to the skillet and cook for 1 minute until fragrant.
3. Sprinkle some salt and pepper on the shrimp before adding them to the pan. Cook until pink and opaque, about 2 to 3 minutes per side.
4. Remove the cooked shrimp from the skillet and set aside.
5. In the same skillet, add the remaining tablespoon of olive oil and the spiralized

zucchini noodles. Cook for 2-3 minutes until tender-crisp.

6. Return the cooked shrimp to the skillet with the zucchini noodles.
7. Drizzle lemon juice over the shrimp and noodles, then toss to combine.
8. Sprinkle chopped fresh parsley over the top.
9. Allow the shrimp scampi with zucchini noodles to cool completely before dividing it into meal prep containers.

Nutrition Value (per serving):
- Calories: 250 kcal
- Protein: 25g
- Carbohydrates: 10g
- Fat: 12g
- Fiber: 3g
- Sugar: 5g
- Sodium: 400mg

Vegetarian Pizza with Whole Wheat Crust and Fresh Vegetables

Preparation time: 15 minutes
Cooking time: 15 minutes
Servings: 4

Ingredients:

- 1 whole wheat pizza crust (store-bought or homemade)
- 1/2 cup pizza sauce
- 1 cup shredded mozzarella cheese
- 1/2 cup sliced bell peppers
- 1/2 cup sliced mushrooms
- 1/4 cup sliced red onion
- 1/4 cup sliced black olives
- 1 tablespoon olive oil
- Salt and pepper to taste
- Optional toppings: fresh basil, crushed red pepper flakes

Directions:

1. Preheat your oven to 425°F (220°C).
2. Place the whole wheat pizza crust on a baking sheet lined with parchment paper.
3. Leaving a thin border all the way around the edges, evenly distribute the pizza sauce over the crust.
4. Sprinkle the shredded mozzarella cheese over the sauce.
5. Arrange the sliced bell peppers, mushrooms, red onion, and black olives on top of the cheese.
6. Drizzle olive oil over the vegetables and season with salt and pepper to taste.

7. Bake in the preheated oven for 12-15 minutes, or until the crust is golden brown and the cheese is melted and bubbly.
8. Remove from the oven and let the pizza cool for a few minutes before slicing.
9. Once cooled, slice the pizza into individual servings and store it in an airtight container in the refrigerator.

Nutrition Value (per serving):
- Calories: 250 kcal
- Protein: 10g
- Carbohydrates: 30g
- Fat: 10g
- Fiber: 5g
- Sugar: 3g
- Sodium: 450mg

Quinoa and Black Bean Stuffed Acorn Squash

Preparation time: 10 minutes
Cooking time: 45 minutes
Servings: 4

Ingredients:
- 2 acorn squashes, halved and seeds removed

- 1 cup quinoa, rinsed
- 2 cups vegetable broth
- 1 can (15 oz) black beans, rinsed and drained
- 1 cup fresh or frozen corn kernels
- 1 teaspoon cumin
- 1/2 teaspoon chilli powder
- Salt and pepper to taste
- Optional toppings: salsa, chopped fresh cilantro

Directions:

1. Preheat the oven to 400°F (200°C).
2. Place the acorn squash halves cut-side down on a baking sheet lined with parchment paper. Bake for 30-35 minutes, or until tender.
3. While the squash is baking, prepare the quinoa. In a medium saucepan, combine the quinoa and vegetable broth. Bring to a boil, then reduce the heat to low, cover, and simmer for 15-20 minutes, or until the quinoa is cooked and the liquid is absorbed.
4. In a large mixing bowl, combine the cooked quinoa, black beans, corn, cumin, chilli powder, salt, and pepper.
5. Once the squash is tender, remove it from the oven and carefully flip the halves over.

6. Spoon the quinoa and black bean mixture into the center of each squash half.
7. Return the stuffed squash to the oven and bake for an additional 10-15 minutes, or until heated through.
8. Allow the stuffed squash to cool completely before storing it in an airtight container in the refrigerator.

Nutrition Value (per serving):
- Calories: 350 kcal
- Protein: 12g
- Carbohydrates: 68g
- Fat: 4g
- Fiber: 10g
- Sugar: 6g
- -Sodium: 580mg

Lemon Garlic Herb Roasted Turkey Breast

Preparation time: 10 minutes
Cooking time: 1 hour
Servings: 4

Ingredients:
- 1 pound turkey breast, boneless and skinless
- 2 tablespoons olive oil

- 2 cloves garlic, minced
- 1 lemon, juiced and zested
- 1 teaspoon dried thyme
- 1 teaspoon dried rosemary
- Salt and pepper to taste

Directions:

1. Preheat the oven to 375°F (190°C).
2. In a small bowl, mix together the olive oil, minced garlic, lemon juice, lemon zest, dried thyme, dried rosemary, salt, and pepper.
3. Place the turkey breast in a baking dish and rub the prepared mixture all over the turkey.
4. Roast the turkey in the preheated oven for 45-60 minutes, or until it reaches an internal temperature of 165°F (75°C).
5. Once cooked, remove the turkey breast from the oven and let it rest for 5-10 minutes before slicing.
6. Slice the turkey breast and divide it into meal prep containers.
7. Allow the turkey to cool completely before storing it in the refrigerator in an airtight container.

Nutrition Value (per serving):

- Calories: 200 kcal
- Protein: 25g

- Carbohydrates: 2g
- Fat: 10g
- Fiber: 0g
- Sugar: 0g
- Sodium: 250mg

Cauliflower Crust Margherita Pizza with Fresh Basil

Preparation time: 15 minutes
Cooking time: 20 minutes
Servings: 2

Ingredients:

- 1 small head cauliflower, riced (about 2 cups)
- 1 egg
- 1/2 cup shredded mozzarella cheese
- 1/4 teaspoon dried oregano
- Salt and pepper to taste
- 1/4 cup tomato sauce
- 1 small tomato, sliced
- 1/4 cup shredded mozzarella cheese
- Fresh basil leaves for garnish

Directions:

1. Preheat your oven to 400°F (200°C). Line a baking sheet with parchment paper.

2. In a microwave-safe bowl, microwave the riced cauliflower for 5-6 minutes, or until soft. Allow it to cool slightly.

3. In a large mixing bowl, combine the cooked cauliflower, egg, 1/2 cup shredded mozzarella cheese, dried oregano, salt, and pepper. Mix until well combined.

4. Transfer the cauliflower mixture onto the prepared baking sheet and spread it out into a thin, even circle to form the pizza crust.

5. Bake the cauliflower crust in the preheated oven for 15-20 minutes, or until golden brown and firm to the touch.

6. Once the crust is baked, remove it from the oven and spread the tomato sauce evenly over the surface.

7. Arrange the tomato slices on top of the sauce, then sprinkle with the remaining shredded mozzarella cheese.

8. Return the pizza to the oven and bake for an additional 5-7 minutes, or until the cheese is melted and bubbly.

9. Remove the pizza from the oven and garnish with fresh basil leaves before serving.

10. Allow it to cool completely before storing it in an airtight container in the refrigerator.

Nutrition Value (per serving):
- Calories: 180 kcal

- Protein: 12g
- Carbohydrates: 10g
- Fat: 10g
- Fiber: 3g
- Sugar: 4g
- Sodium: 380mg

Chickpea and Spinach Curry with Basmati Rice

Preparation time: 10 minutes
Cooking time: 20 minutes
Servings: 4

Ingredients:
- 1 tablespoon olive oil
- 1 onion, finely chopped
- 2 cloves garlic, minced
- 1 tablespoon curry powder
- 1 teaspoon ground cumin
- 1 teaspoon ground coriander
- 1/2 teaspoon turmeric
- 1 can (15 ounces) chickpeas, drained and rinsed
- 1 can (14 ounces) diced tomatoes
- 2 cups fresh spinach leaves
- Salt and pepper to taste
- 2 cups cooked basmati rice

Directions:

1. Heat olive oil in a large skillet over medium heat. Add and sauté the chopped onion and minced garlic for 2-3 minutes, until softened.
2. Stir in the curry powder, ground cumin, ground coriander, and turmeric, and cook for another 1-2 minutes until fragrant.
3. Add the drained chickpeas and diced tomatoes to the skillet. Stir well to combine.
4. Reduce the heat to low and let the mixture simmer for 10 minutes, allowing the flavours to meld together.
5. Add the fresh spinach leaves to the skillet and cook for an additional 2-3 minutes until wilted.
6. Season with pepper and salt to taste.
7. Divide the cooked basmati rice into meal prep containers.
8. Spoon the chickpea and spinach curry over the rice, dividing it evenly among the containers.
9. Allow the curry to cool completely before sealing the containers and storing them in the refrigerator.

Nutrition Value (per serving):

- Calories: 350 kcal
- Protein: 12g

- Carbohydrates: 60g
- Fat: 7g
- Fiber: 10g
- Sugar: 5g
- Sodium: 480mg

Baked Eggplant Parmesan Stacks with Tomato Sauce and Mozzarella

Preparation time: 15 minutes
Cooking time: 30 minutes
Servings: 2

Ingredients:
- 1 medium eggplant, sliced into rounds
- 1 cup marinara sauce
- 1 cup shredded mozzarella cheese
- 1/4 cup grated Parmesan cheese
- 1 teaspoon dried Italian seasoning
- Salt and pepper to taste
- Olive oil spray

Directions:
1. Preheat the oven to 400°F (200°C).
2. Arrange the eggplant slices on a baking sheet lined with parchment paper. Spray

both sides of the eggplant slices with olive oil spray and season with salt and pepper.

3. Bake the eggplant slices for 15-20 minutes, flipping halfway through, until tender and lightly golden brown.

4. Remove the baking sheet from the oven and reduce the oven temperature to 350°F (180°C).

5. In a small bowl, mix together the marinara sauce and dried Italian seasoning.

6. To assemble the stacks, place a baked eggplant slice on a baking dish. Top with a spoonful of marinara sauce, a sprinkle of shredded mozzarella cheese, and a sprinkle of grated Parmesan cheese. Repeat the layers until all the eggplant slices are used, finishing with a layer of cheese on top.

7. Bake the eggplant stacks in the preheated oven for 10-12 minutes, or until the cheese is melted and bubbly.

8. Allow to cool completely before storing them in an airtight container in the refrigerator.

Nutrition Value (per serving):
- Calories: 280 kcal
- Protein: 16g
- Carbohydrates: 20g
- Fat: 15g

- Fiber: 8g
- Sugar: 10g
- Sodium: 550mg

Lemon Garlic Shrimp Pasta with Whole Wheat Linguine

Preparation time: 10 minutes
Cooking time: 15 minutes
Servings: 4

Ingredients:
- 8 ounces whole wheat linguine
- 1 pound shrimp, peeled and deveined
- 4 cloves garlic, minced
- 2 tablespoons olive oil
- 1 lemon, juiced and zested
- Salt and pepper to taste
- 2 tablespoons chopped fresh parsley

Directions:
1. Cook the whole wheat linguine according to package instructions. Drain and set aside.
2. In a large skillet, heat olive oil over medium heat. Add and cook minced garlic until fragrant, for about 1 minute.
3. Add shrimp to the skillet and cook until pink and opaque, about 2-3 minutes per side.

4. Add cooked linguine to the skillet with the shrimp and garlic.
5. Pour lemon juice over the pasta and shrimp, then sprinkle lemon zest on top.
6. Season with salt and pepper to taste, and toss everything together until well combined.
7. Divide the lemon garlic shrimp pasta into meal prep containers.
8. Garnish each serving with chopped fresh parsley.
9. Allow the pasta to cool completely before storing it in the refrigerator.

Nutrition Value (per serving):
- Calories: 350 kcal
- Protein: 25g
- Carbohydrates: 40g
- Fat: 10g
- Fiber: 6g
- Sugar: 2g
- Sodium: 150mg

Turkey Meatball Subs with Whole Wheat Hoagie Rolls and Marinara Sauce

Preparation time: 15 minutes
Cooking time: 20 minutes

Servings: 4

Ingredients:
- 1 pound lean ground turkey
- 1/4 cup breadcrumbs
- 1 egg
- 1/4 cup grated Parmesan cheese
- 1 teaspoon Italian seasoning
- Salt and pepper to taste
- 4 whole wheat hoagie rolls
- 1 cup marinara sauce
- Optional toppings: shredded mozzarella cheese, sliced bell peppers, sliced onions

Directions:
1. Preheat the oven to 375°F (190°C). Line a baking sheet with parchment paper.
2. In a large mixing bowl, combine the ground turkey, breadcrumbs, egg, Parmesan cheese, Italian seasoning, salt, and pepper. Mix until well combined.
3. Shape the turkey mixture into meatballs, about 1 inch in diameter, and place them on the prepared baking sheet.
4. Bake the meatballs in the preheated oven for 15-20 minutes, or until cooked through and lightly browned.

5. While the meatballs are baking, heat the marinara sauce in a saucepan over medium heat until warmed through.
6. Slice the hoagie rolls in half lengthwise, but do not separate completely.
7. Once the meatballs are cooked, place 3-4 meatballs inside each hoagie roll.
8. Spoon marinara sauce over the meatballs and top with optional toppings if desired.
9. Allow the subs to cool completely before storing them in an airtight container in the refrigerator.

Nutrition Value (per serving):
- Calories: 380 kcal
- Protein: 28g
- Carbohydrates: 38g
- Fat: 12g
- Fiber: 6g
- Sugar: 5g
- Sodium: 740mg

Moroccan Vegetable Tagine with Couscous

Preparation time: 15 minutes
Cooking time: 30 minutes
Servings: 4

Ingredients:

- 1 tablespoon olive oil
- 1 onion, chopped
- 2 cloves garlic, minced
- 2 carrots, peeled and diced
- 1 zucchini, diced
- 1 bell pepper, diced
- 1 can (14 oz) diced tomatoes
- 1 can (15 oz) chickpeas, drained and rinsed
- 1 cup vegetable broth
- 1 teaspoon ground cumin
- 1 teaspoon ground coriander
- 1/2 teaspoon ground cinnamon
- Salt and pepper to taste
- 1 cup couscous
- For garnishing: chopped fresh parsley or cilantro

Directions:

1. In a big pot or Dutch oven, warm up the olive oil over medium heat. Add chopped onion and minced garlic. Cook until softened, about 3-4 minutes.
2. Add diced carrots, zucchini, and bell pepper to the pot. Cook for another five minutes, stirring now and then.
3. Stir in diced tomatoes, chickpeas, vegetable broth, ground cumin, ground coriander, ground cinnamon, salt, and pepper. Bring to

a simmer and cook for 15-20 minutes, or until the vegetables are tender.

4. While the tagine is simmering, prepare the couscous according to package instructions.

5. Allow the Moroccan vegetable tagine and couscous to cool completely before storing them in an airtight container in the refrigerator.

Nutrition Value (per serving):

- Calories: 320 kcal
- Protein: 10g
- Carbohydrates: 60g
- Fat: 5g
- Fiber: 10g
- Sugar: 10g
- Sodium: 600mg

Conclusion

In wrapping up our exploration of the DASH (Dietary Approaches to Stop Hypertension) diet and its transformative potential, it's evident that this approach to eating offers far-reaching benefits for overall health and well-being. Throughout this book, we've delved into a rich array of flavorful recipes, carefully crafted to align with the core principles of the DASH diet, emphasizing whole foods, lean proteins, and nutrient-dense ingredients while minimizing sodium and unhealthy fats.

As you navigate your culinary journey with the DASH diet, it's essential to extend your commitment to healthy eating beyond the confines of your home kitchen. When dining out, maintain a discerning eye for menu options that mirror the wholesome ethos of the DASH diet. Seek out establishments that prioritize fresh, minimally processed ingredients and don't hesitate to request modifications to accommodate your dietary preferences.

Moreover, let's not overlook the pivotal role of regular physical activity in fortifying the benefits of the DASH diet. By integrating exercise into your daily routine, you amplify the positive impact of your dietary choices, fostering cardiovascular health, enhancing metabolic function, and bolstering overall vitality. Aim for a balanced regimen that incorporates both aerobic exercise and strength training to maximize your fitness potential.

As you embark on your journey towards a healthier lifestyle, remember to approach each day with intentionality, mindfulness, and a steadfast commitment to your well-being. By embracing the principles of the DASH diet, adopting a proactive stance towards dining out, and incorporating regular exercise into your routine, you're forging a path towards sustained health and vitality.

Here's to a future brimming with vitality, nourishment, and fulfilment. Cheers to your continued success on this journey towards optimal health!

www.ingramcontent.com/pod-product-compliance
Lightning Source LLC
Chambersburg PA
CBHW050807260726
48660CB00004B/1292